I0116408

Mythical Creatures Coloring Book

Aryla Publishing 2020

978-1-912675-85-2

www.arylapublishing.com

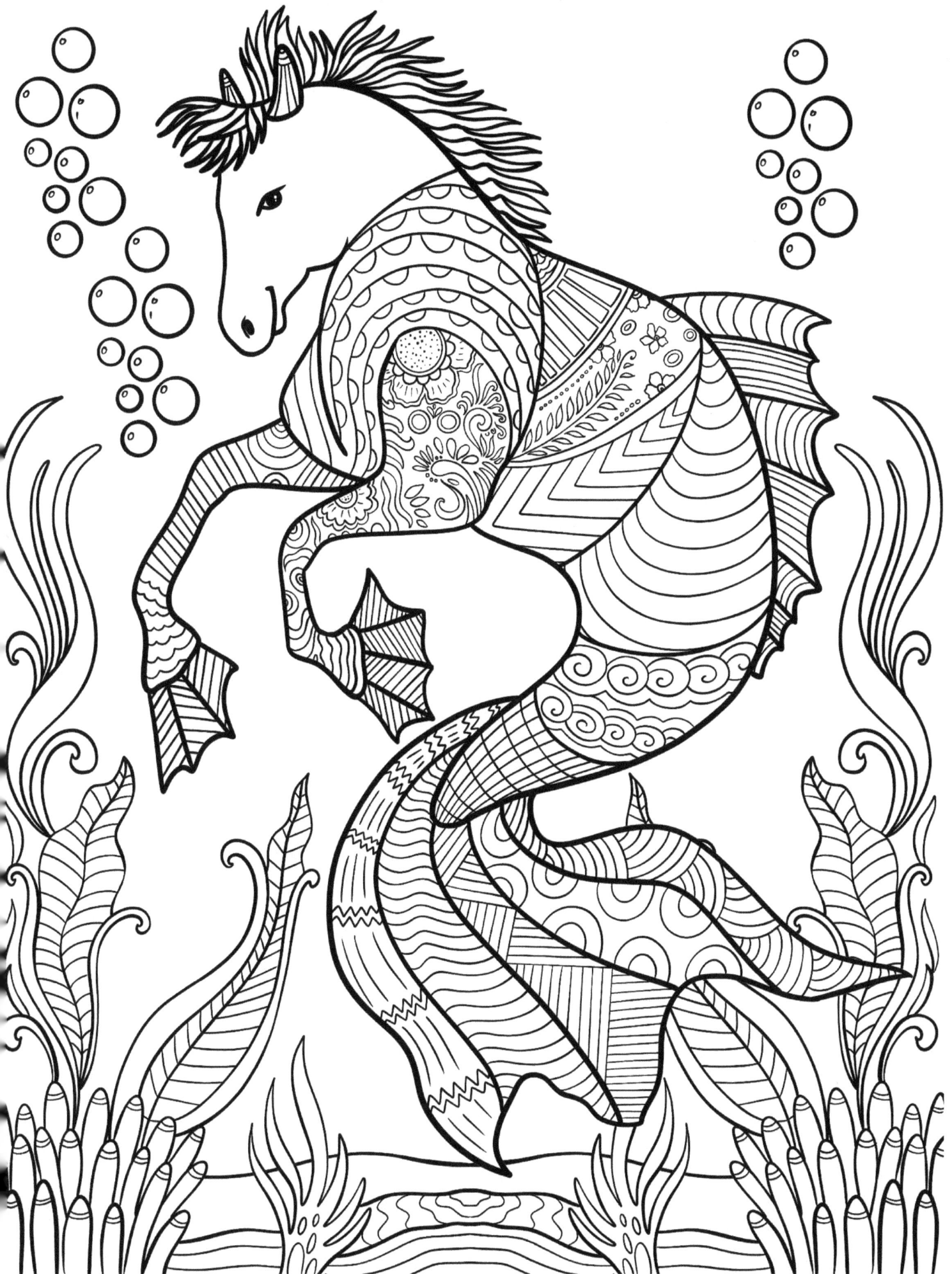

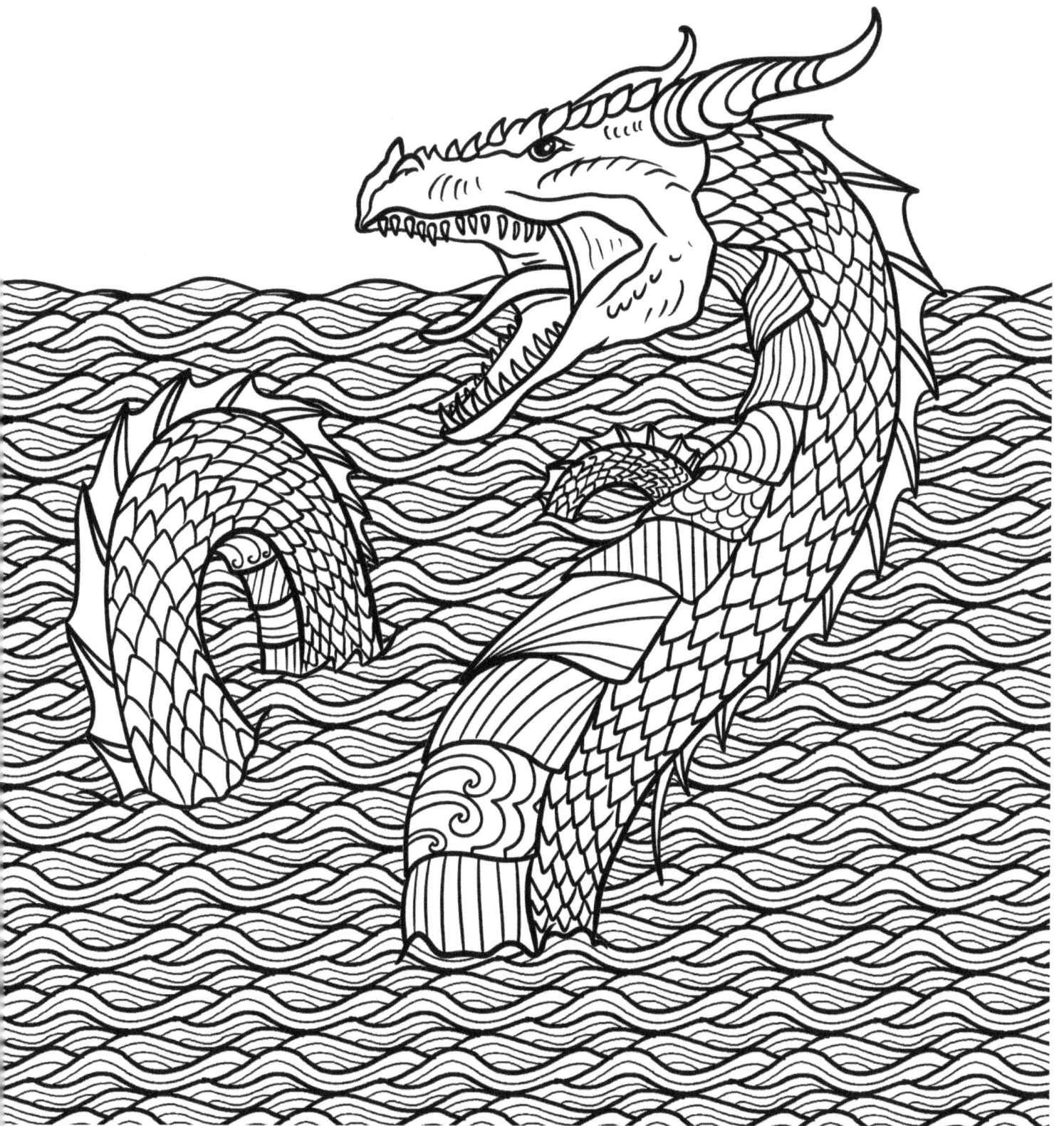

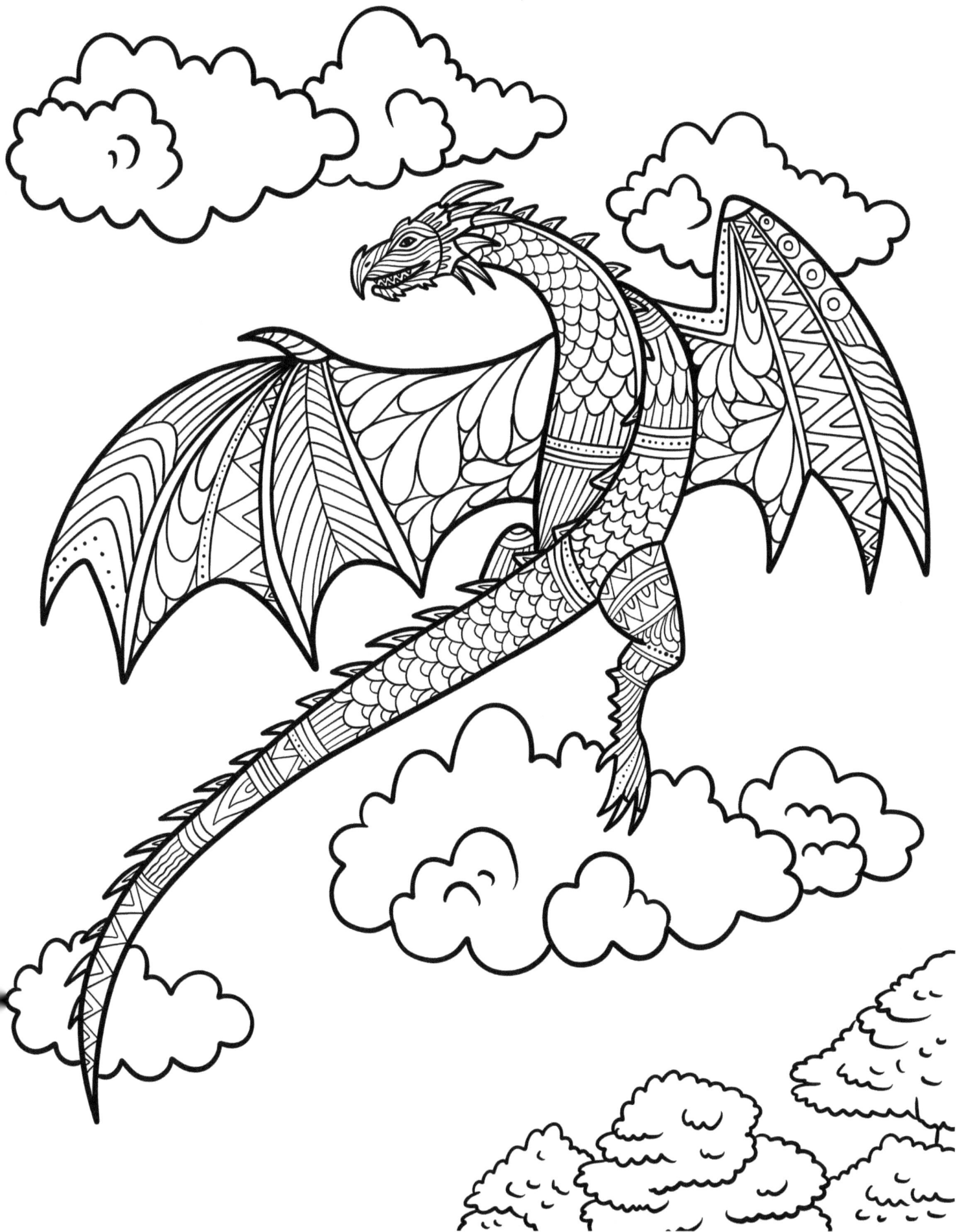

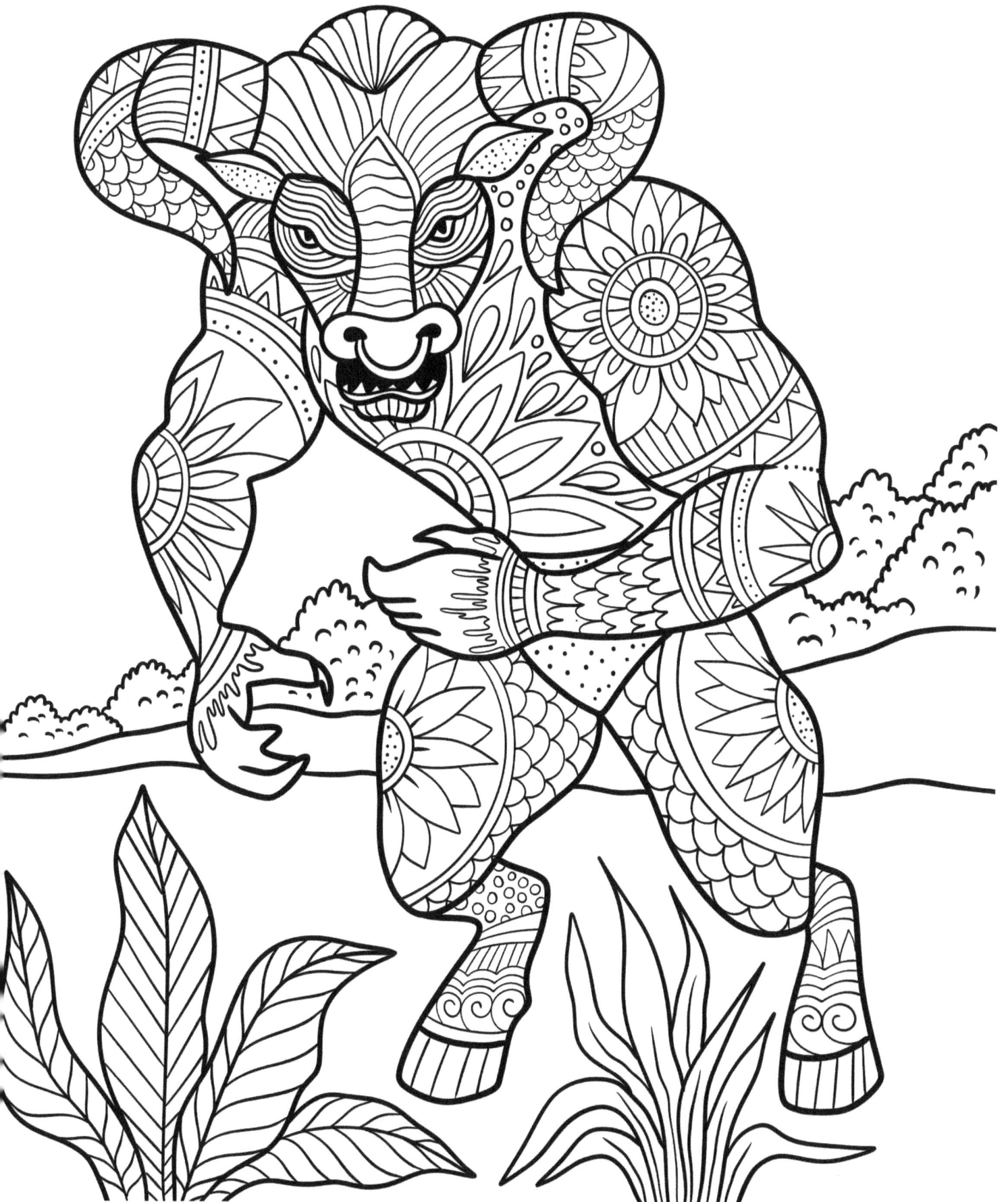

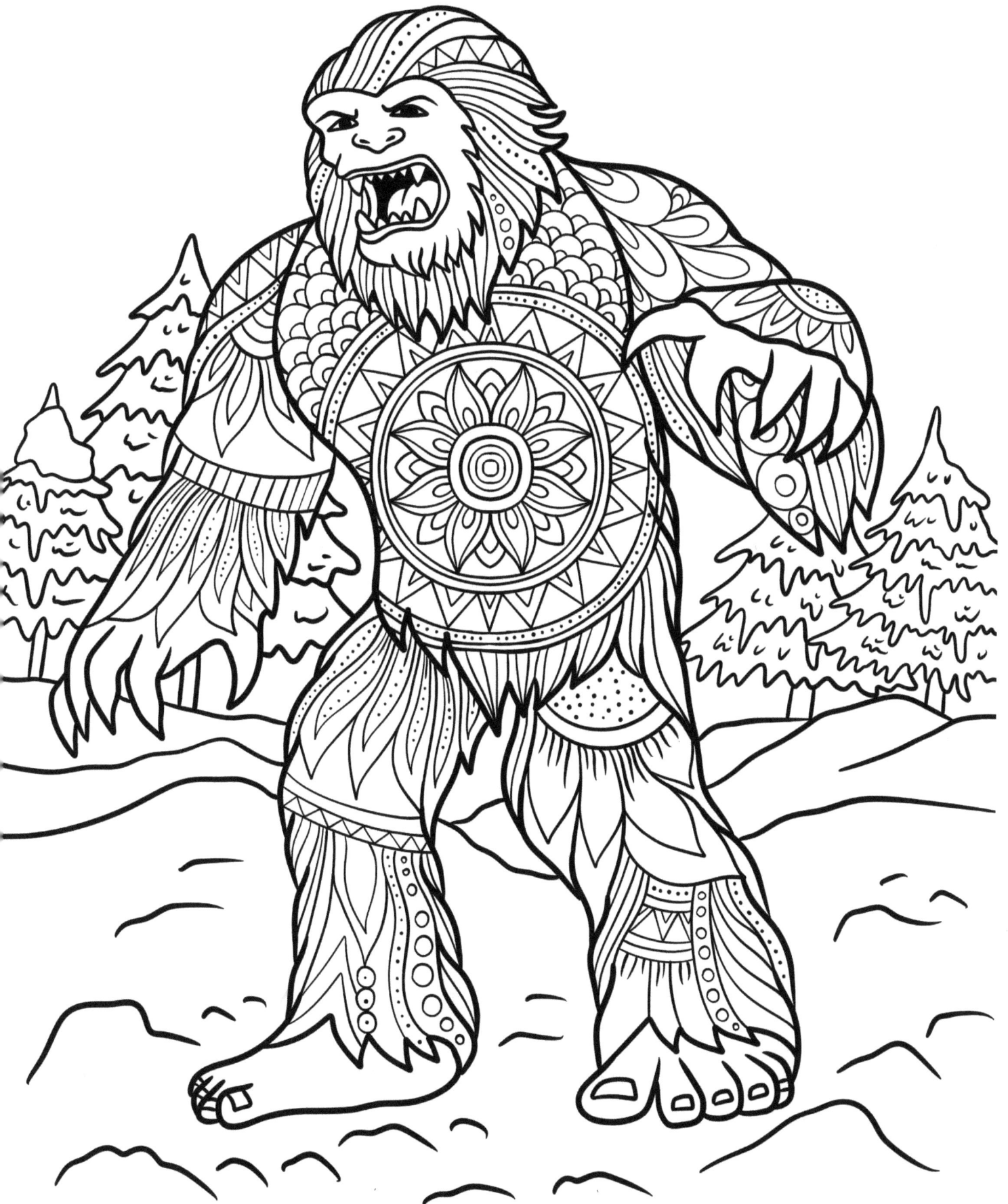

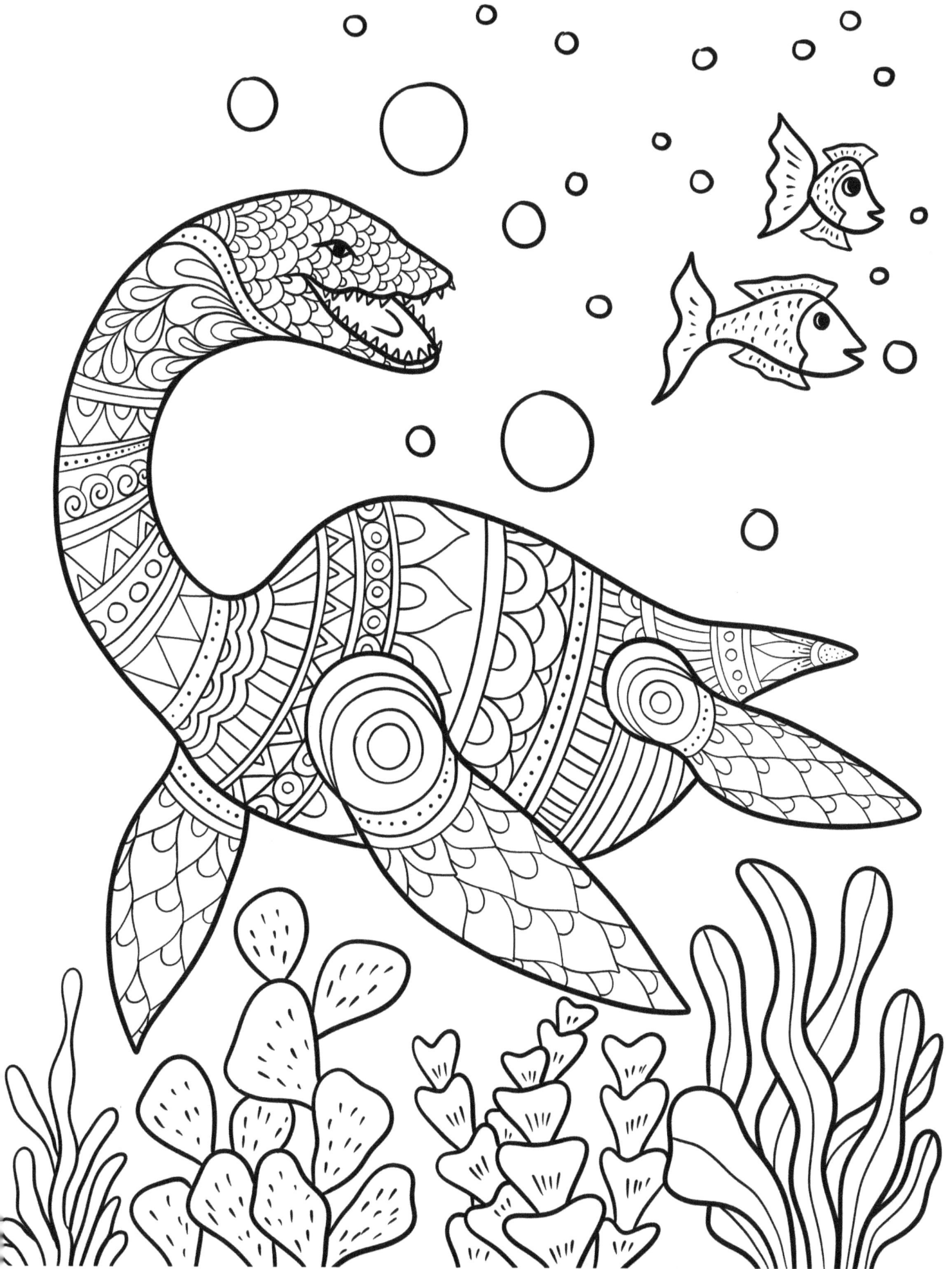

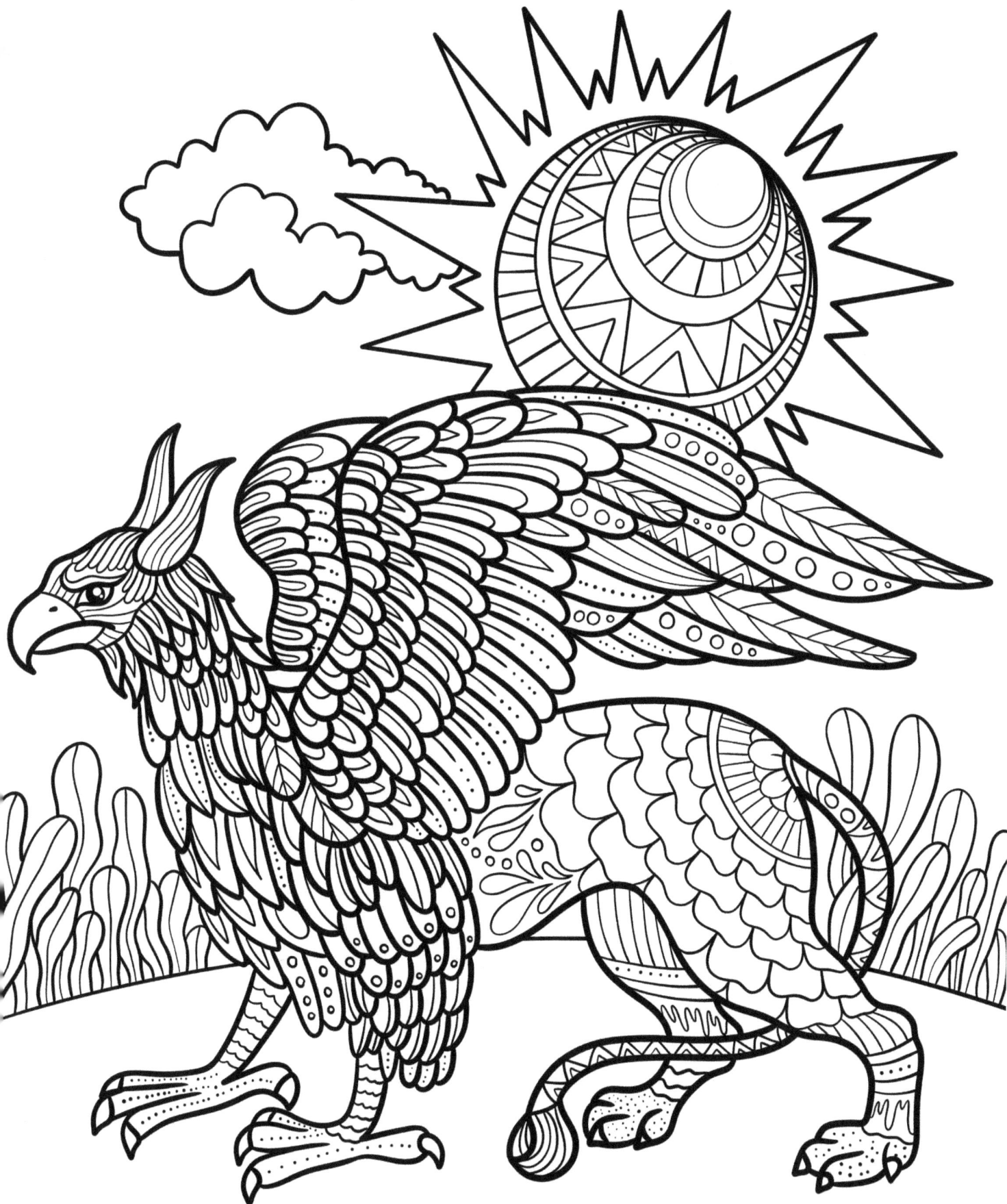

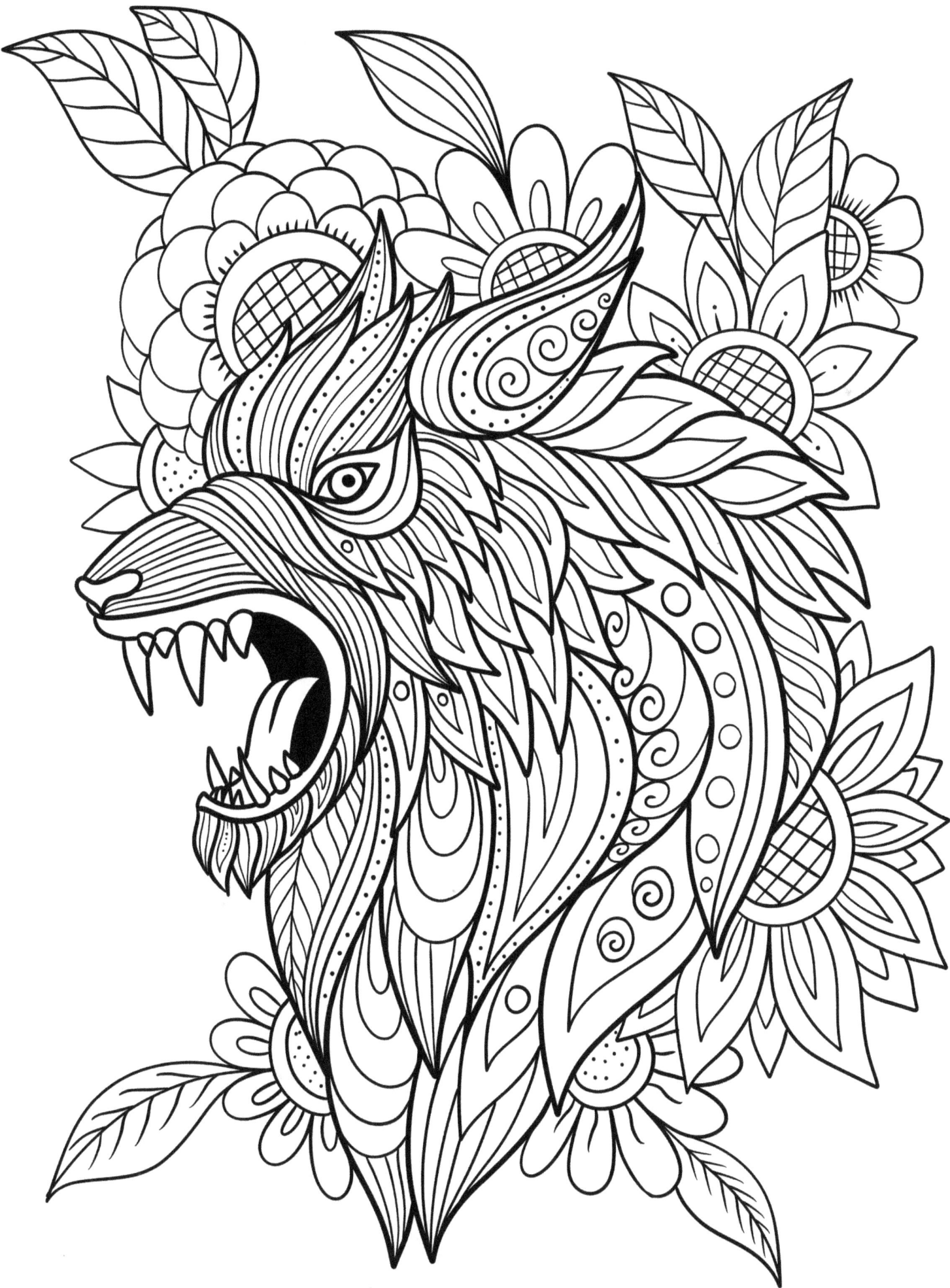

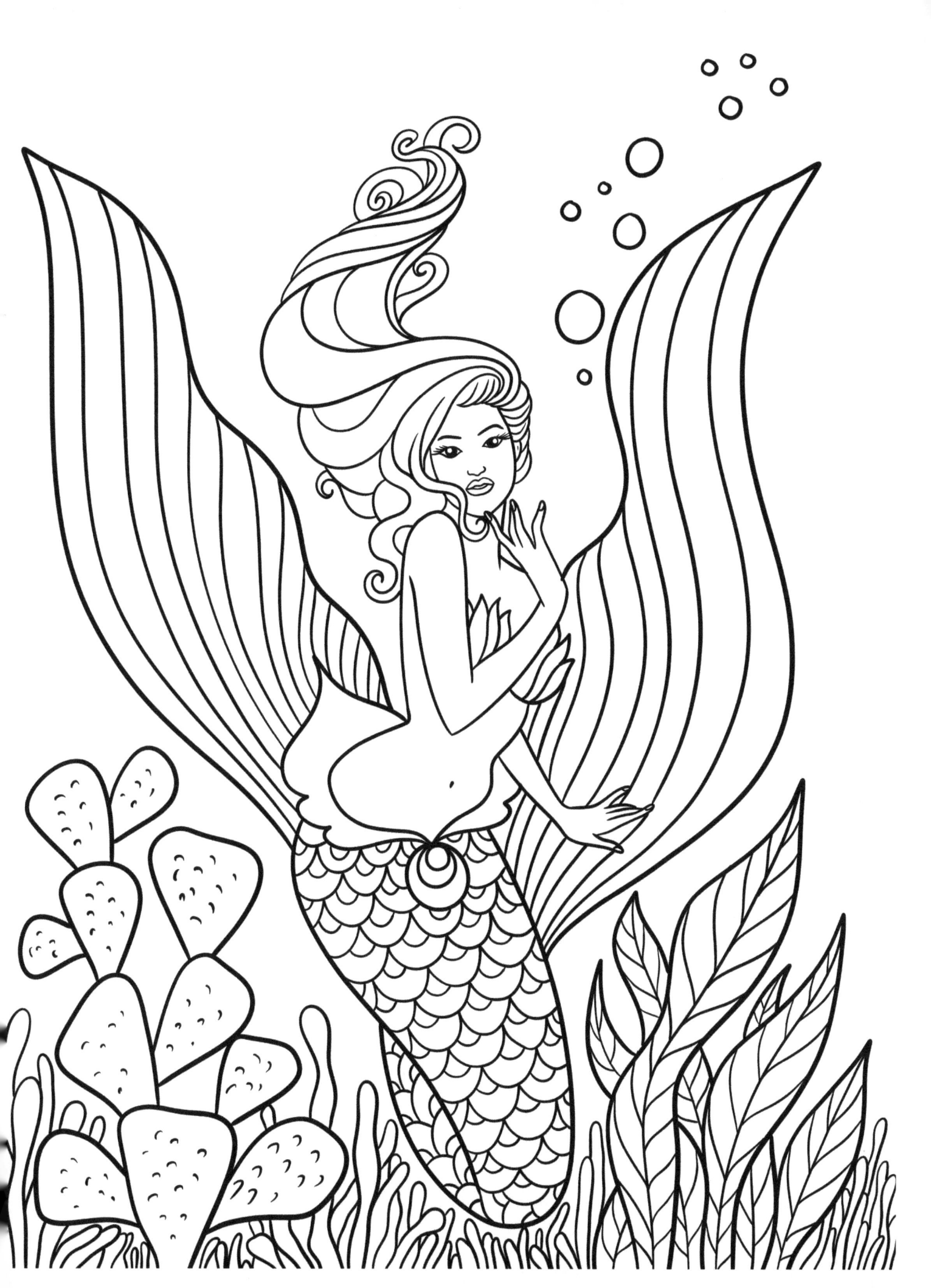

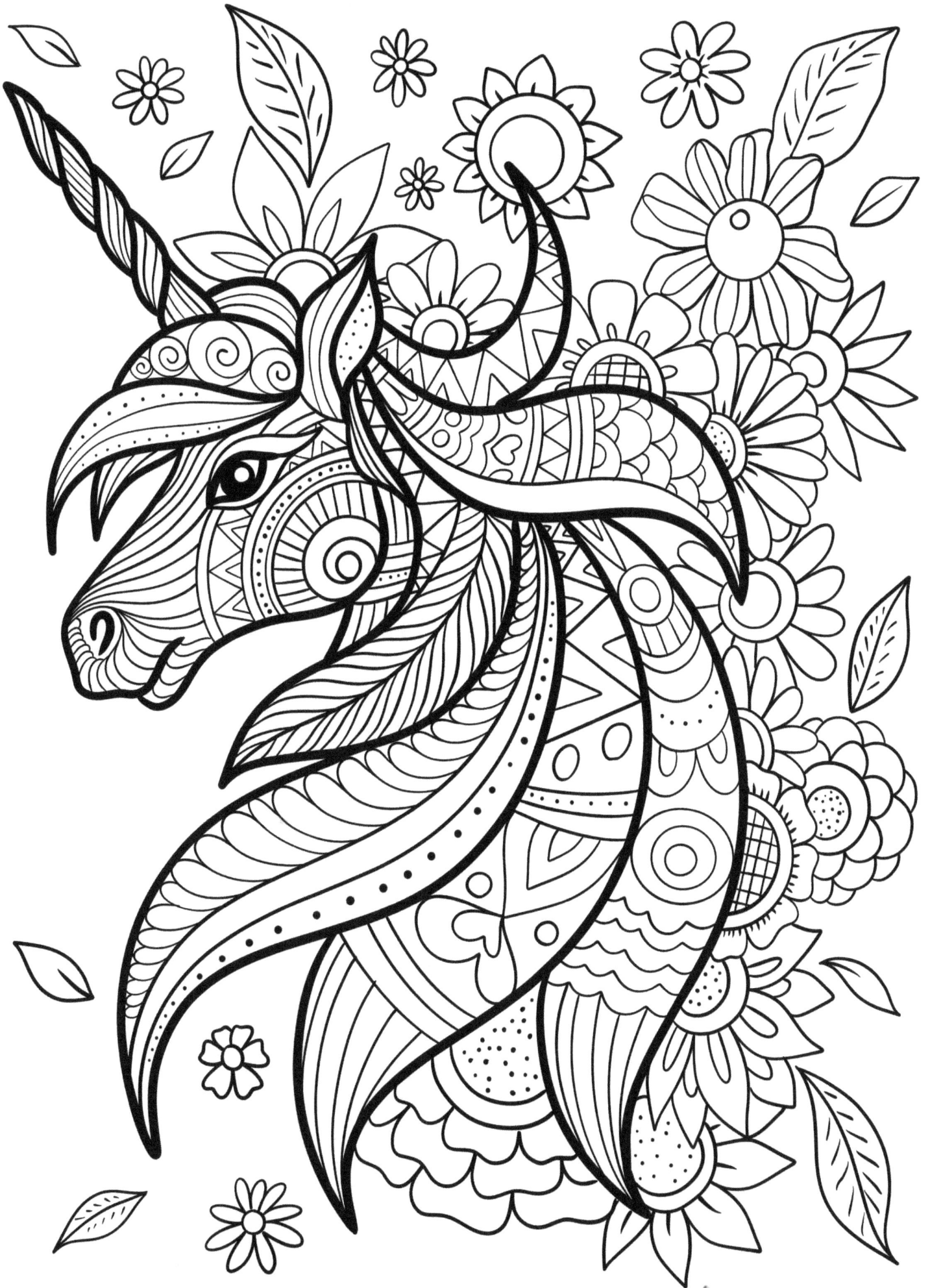

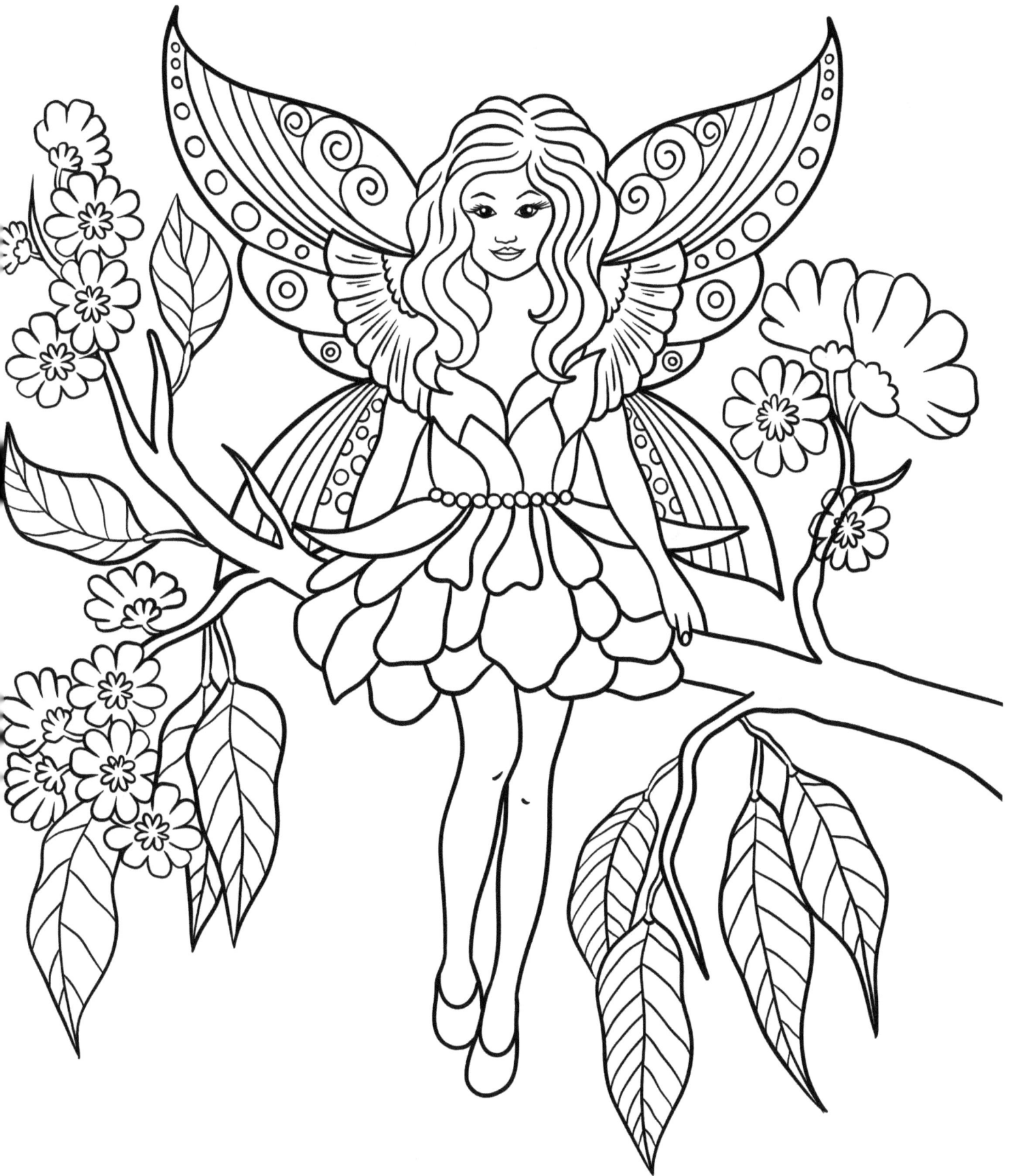

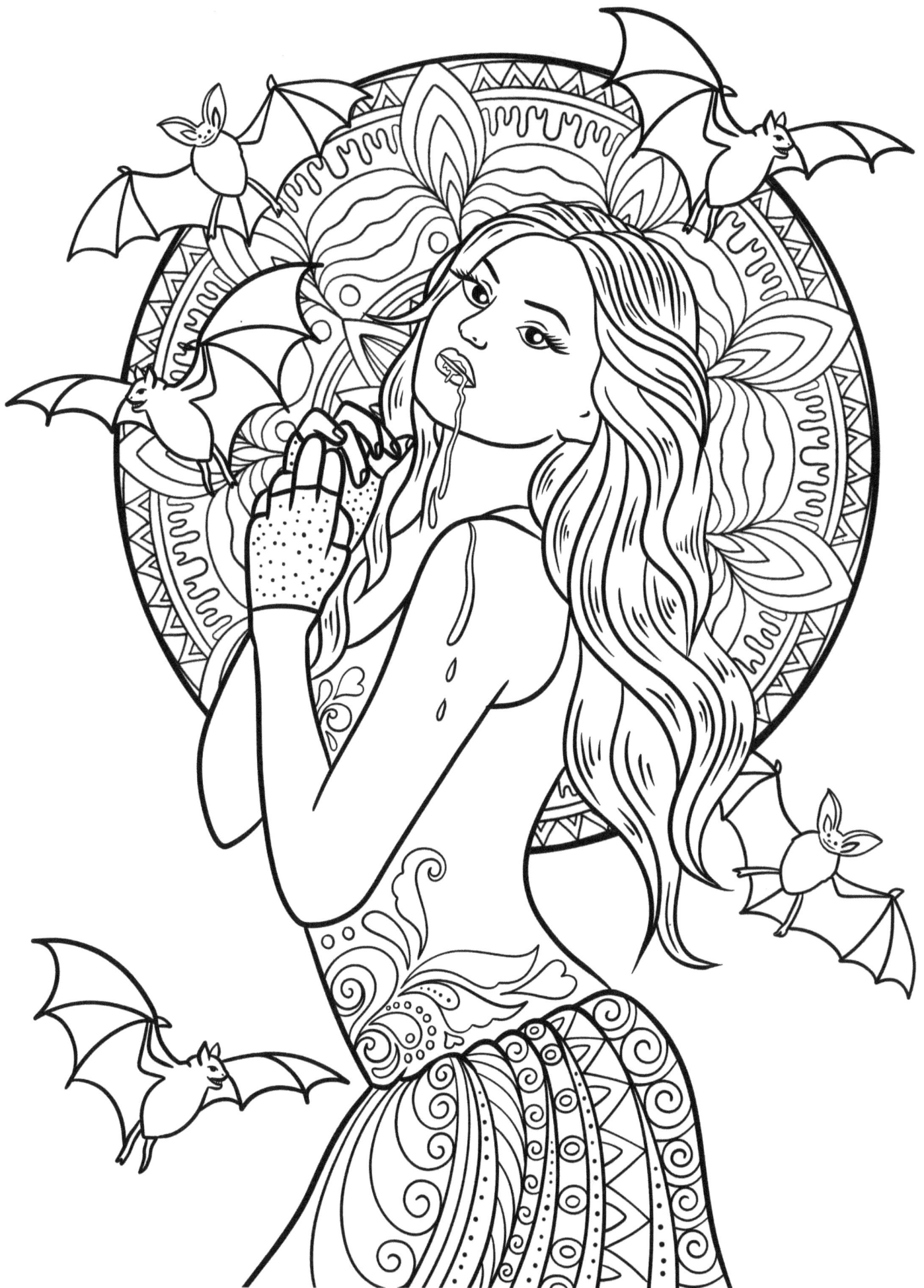

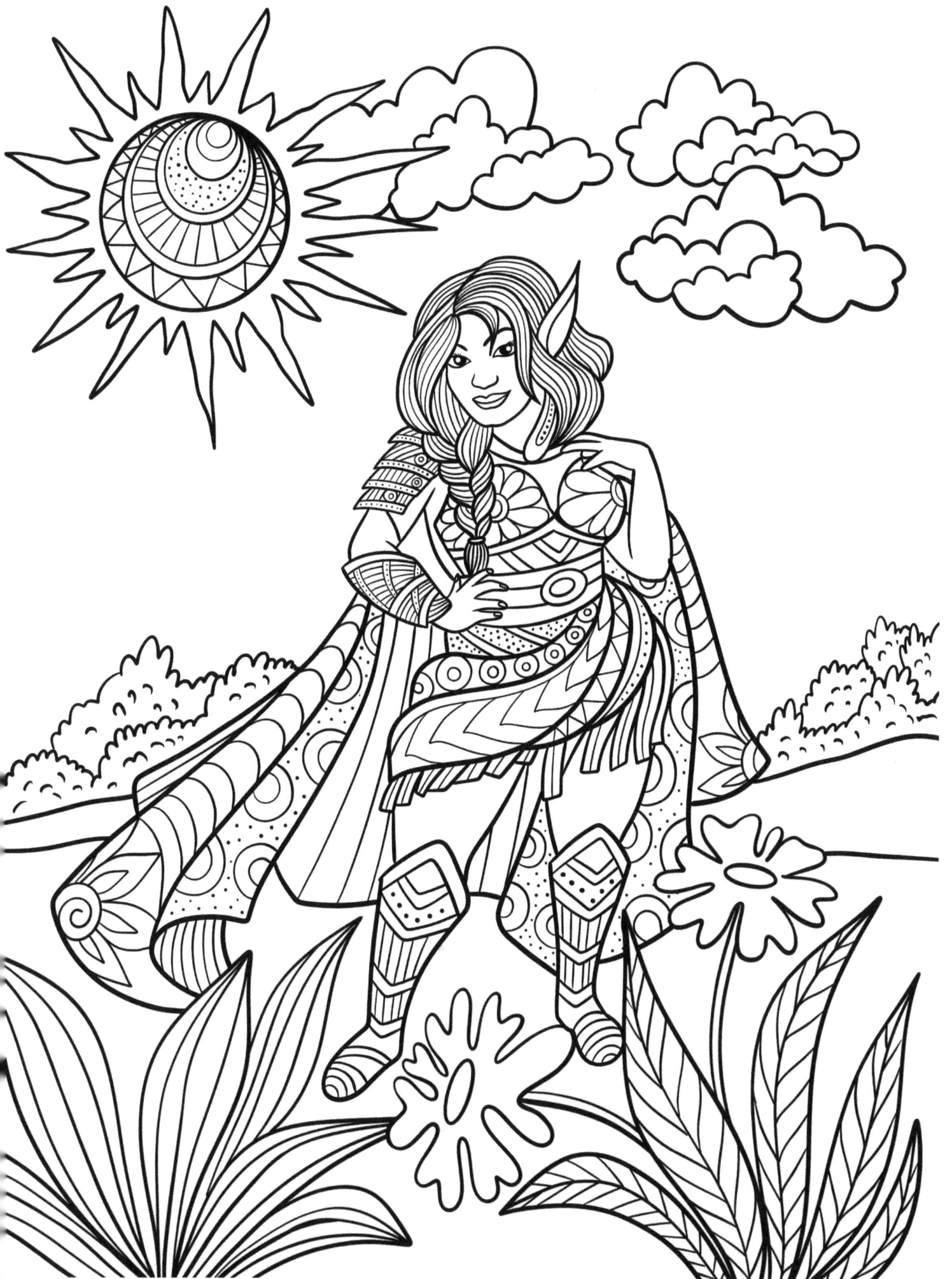

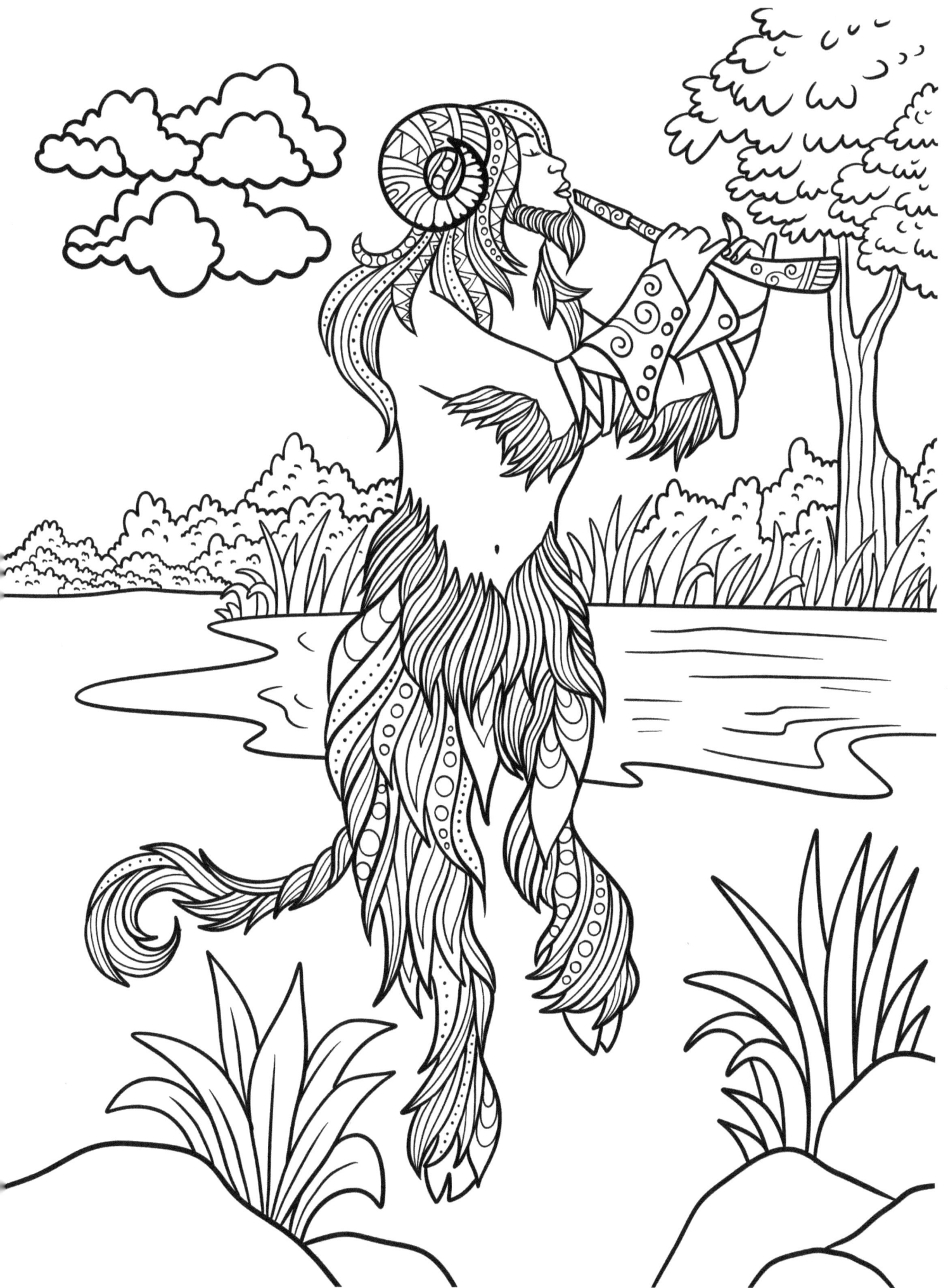

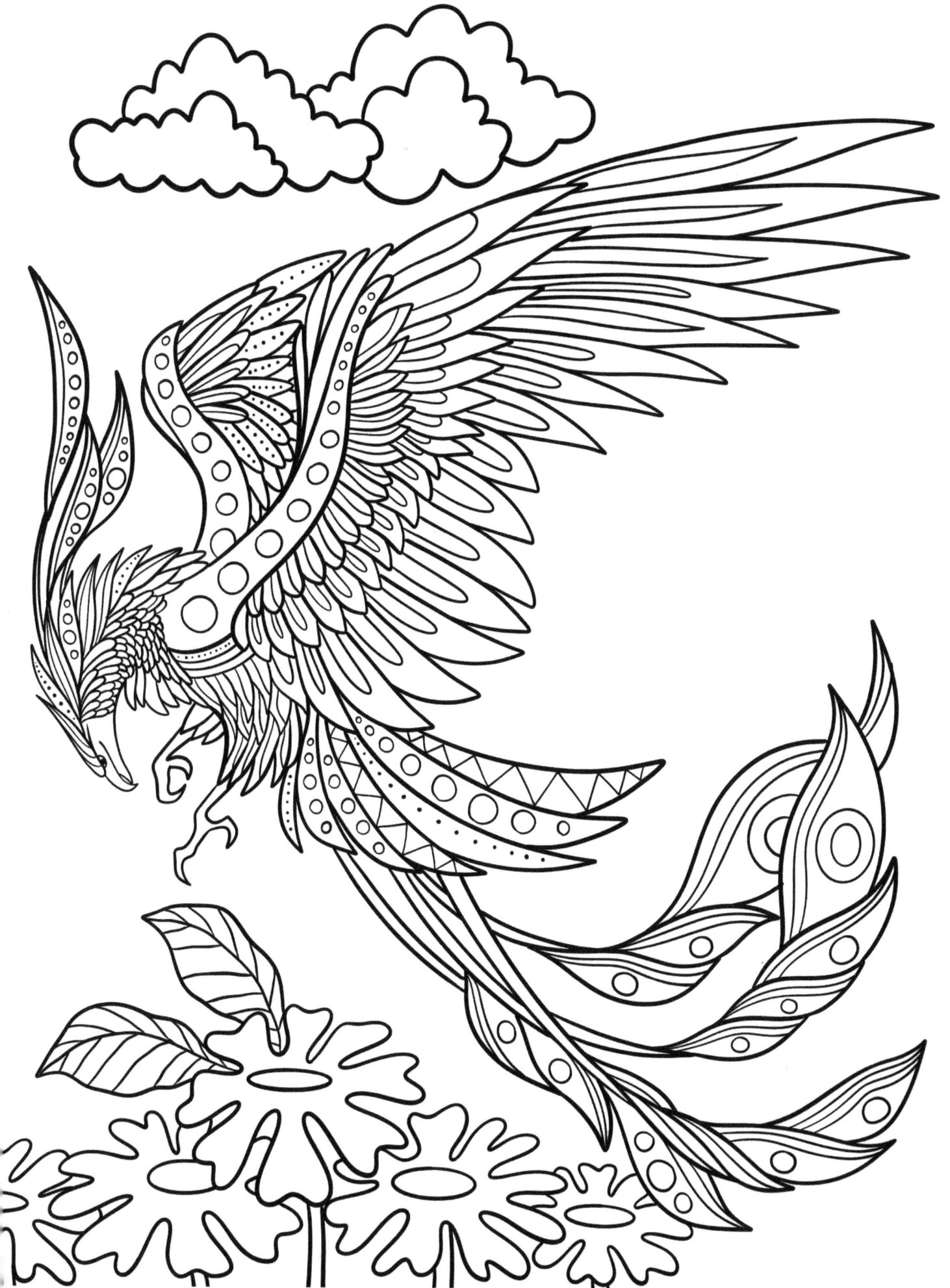

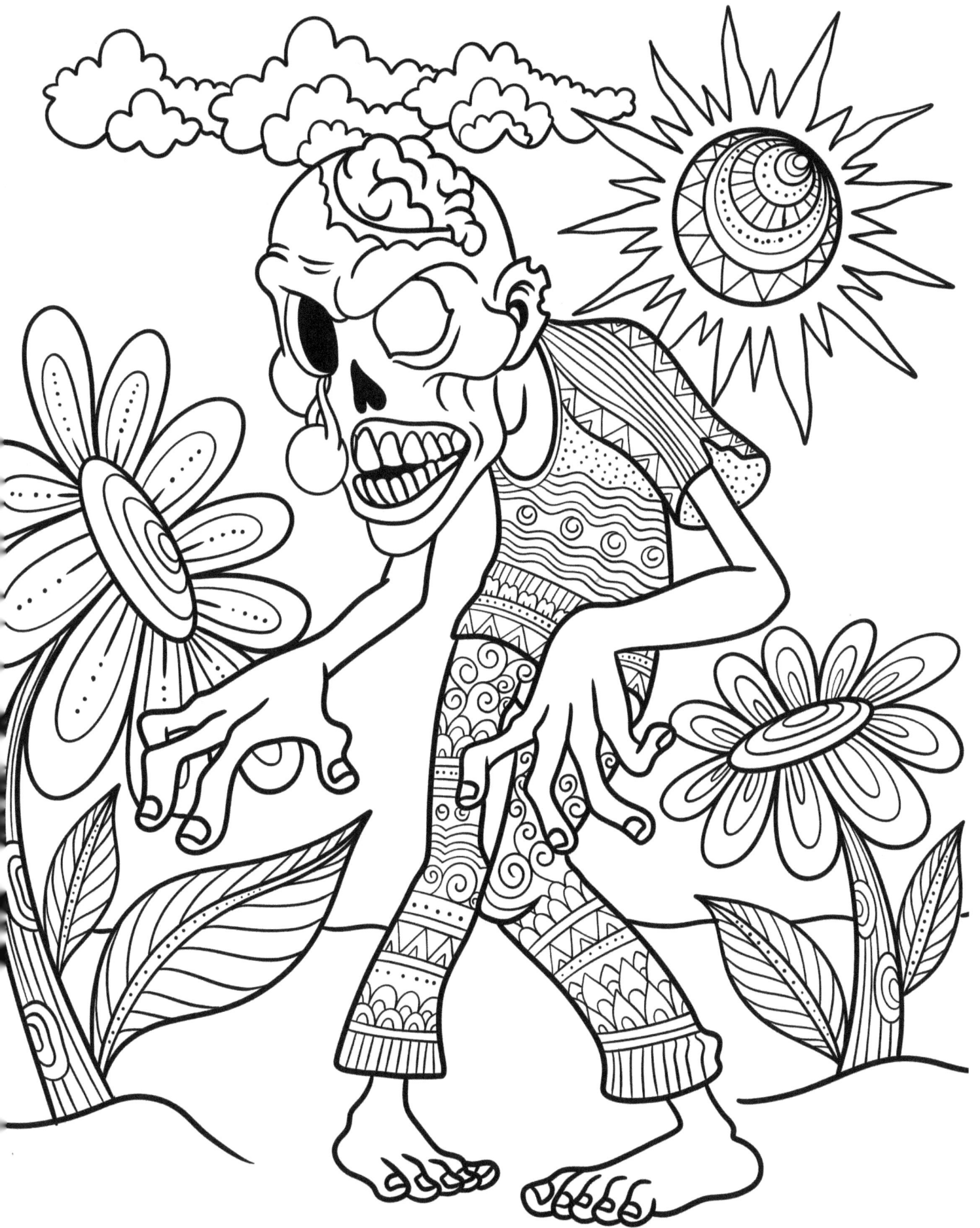

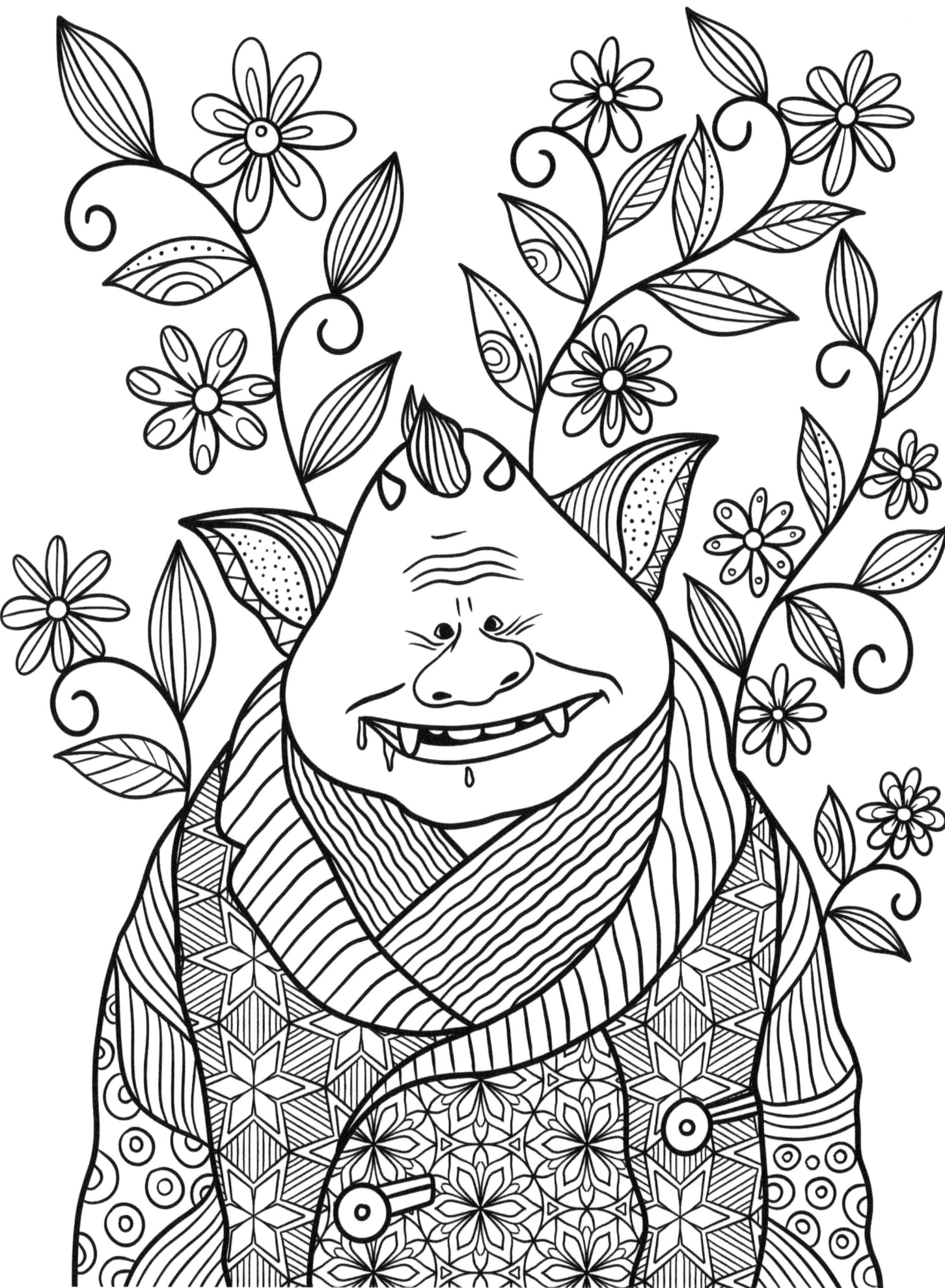

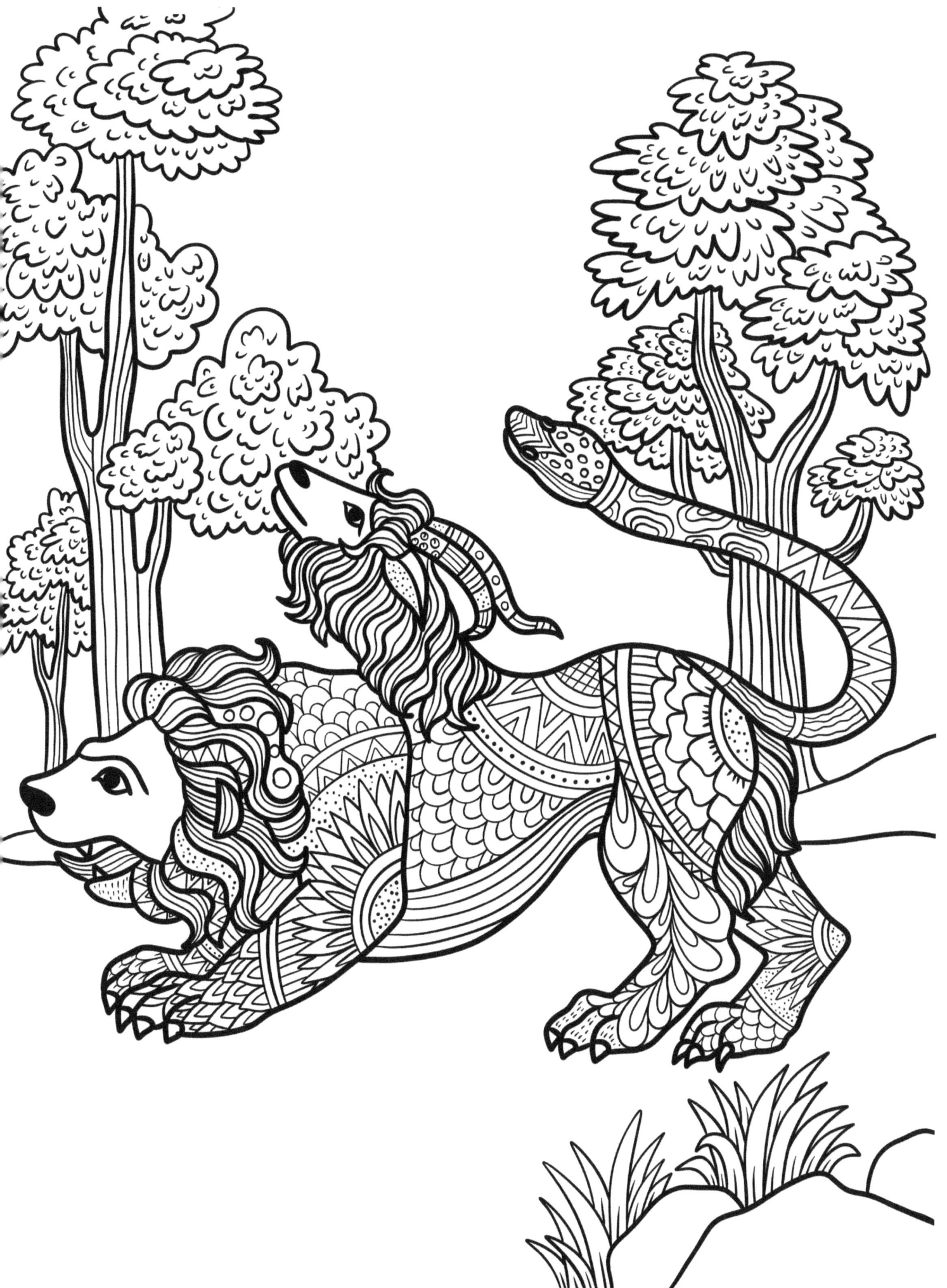

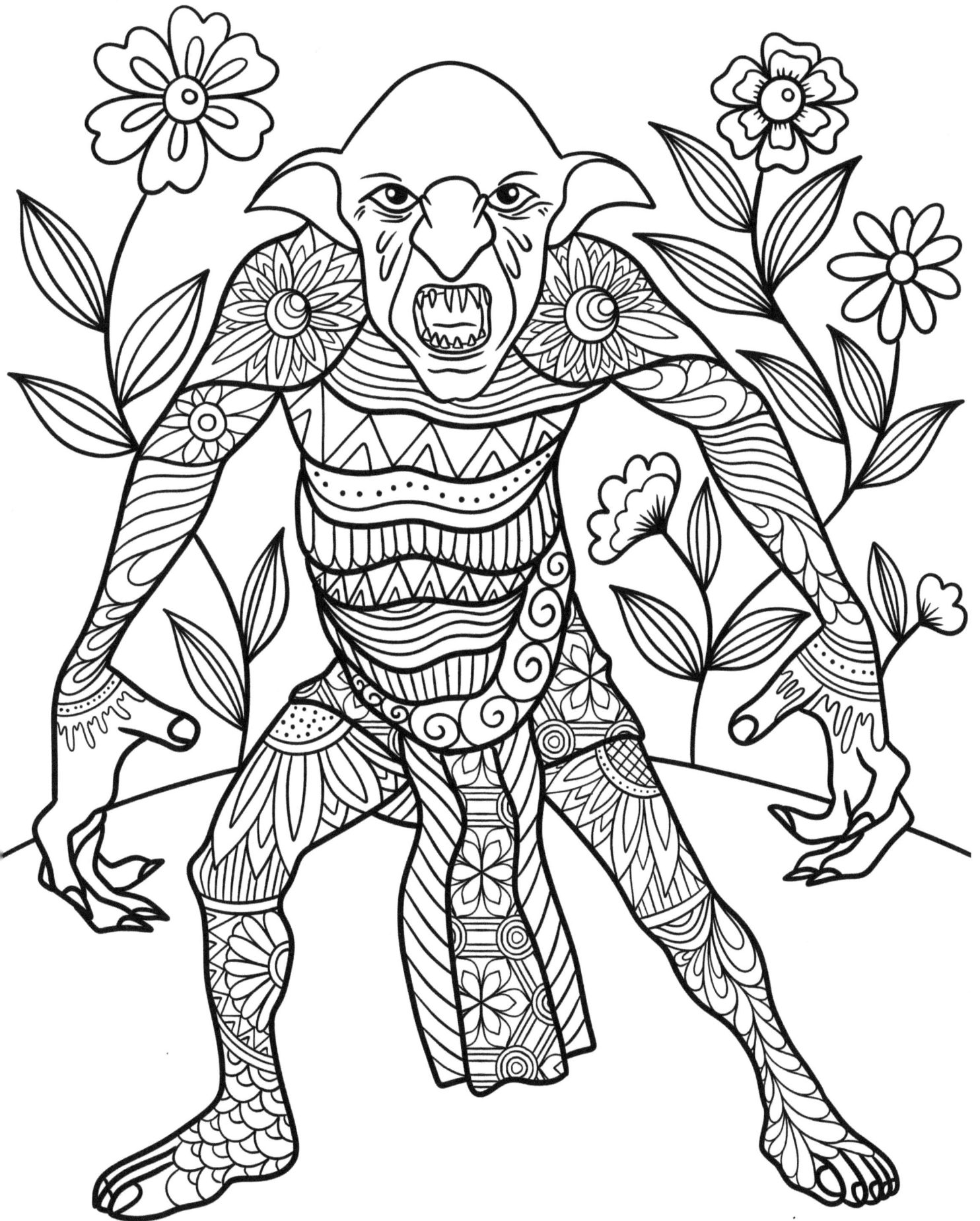

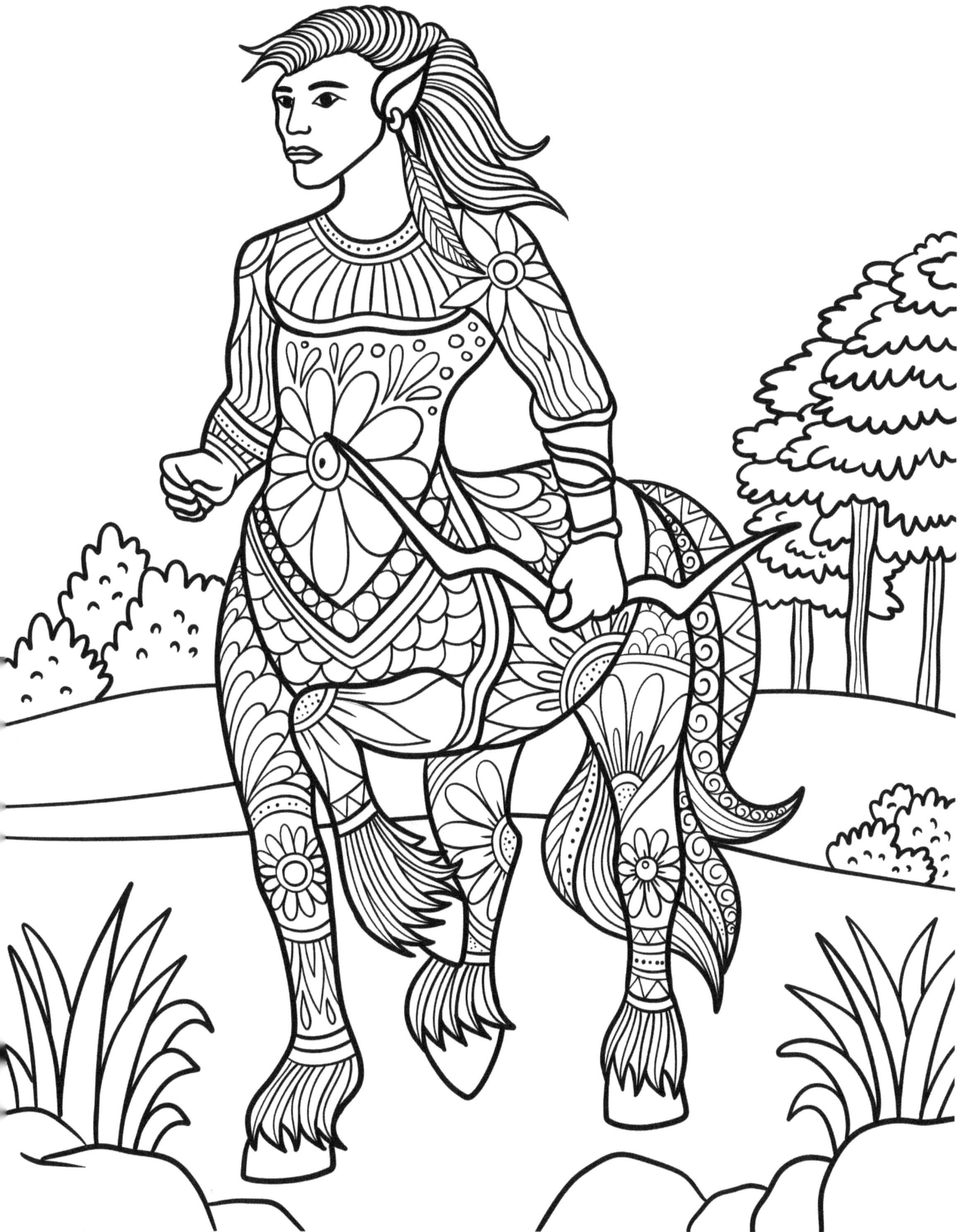

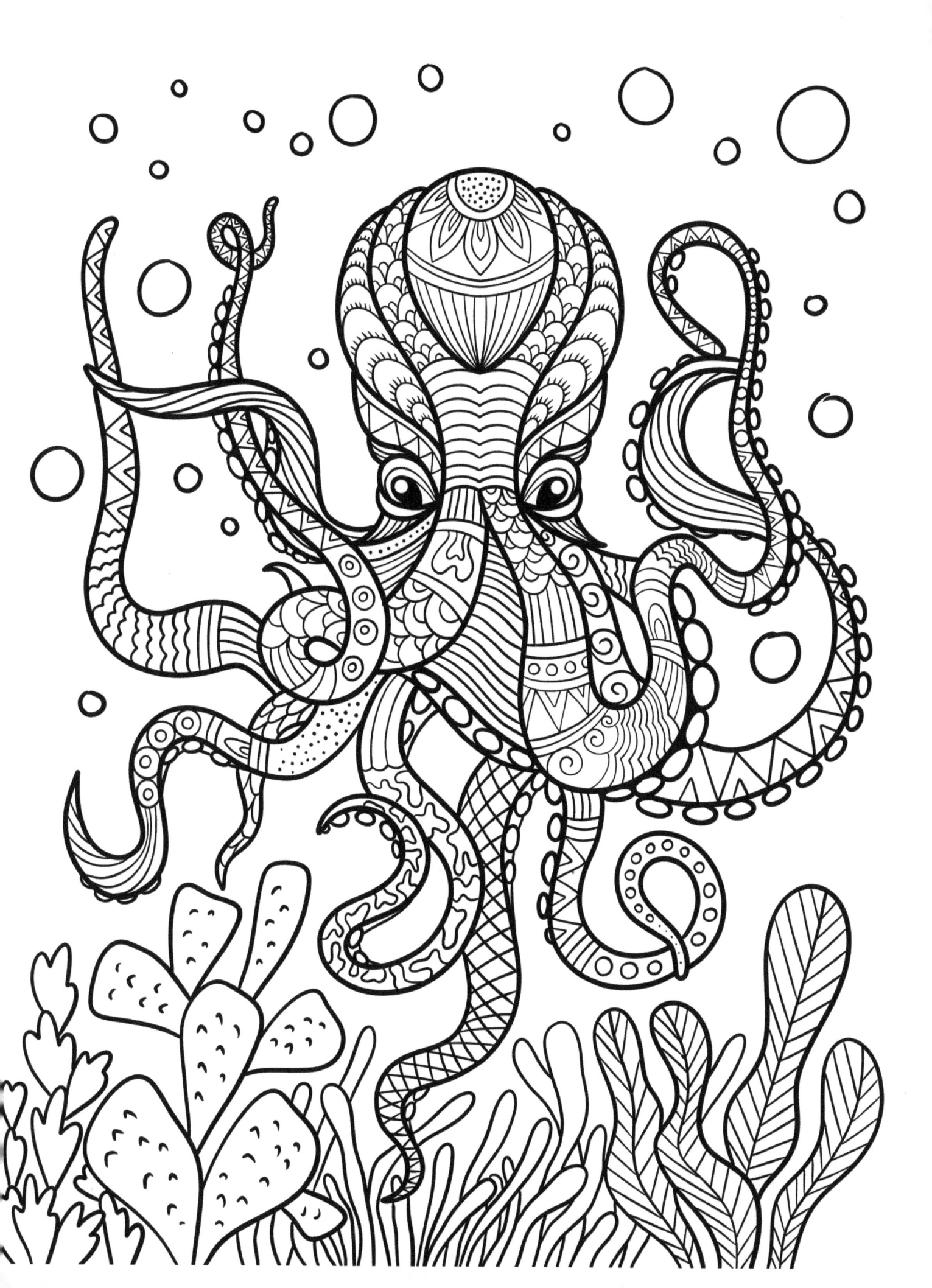

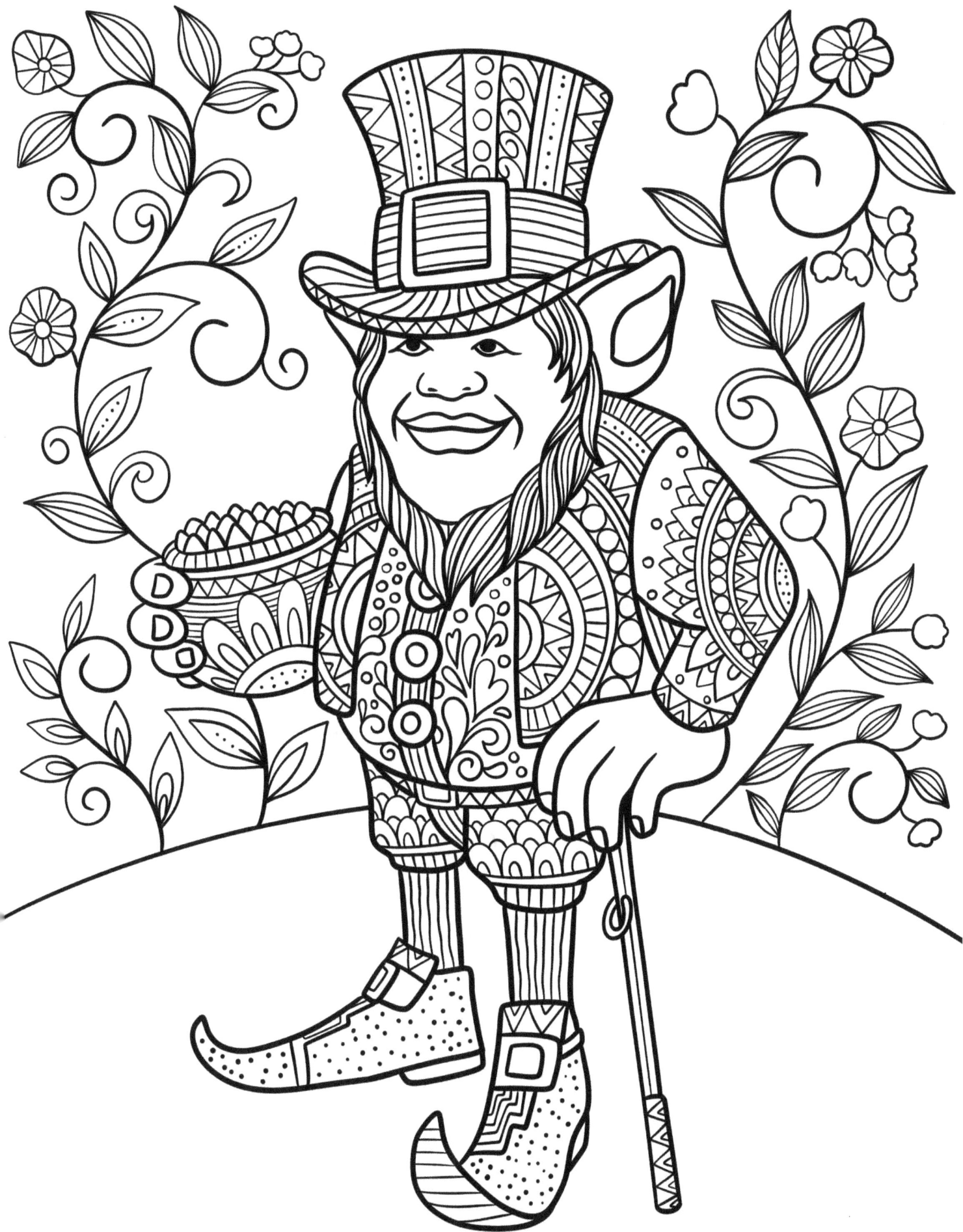

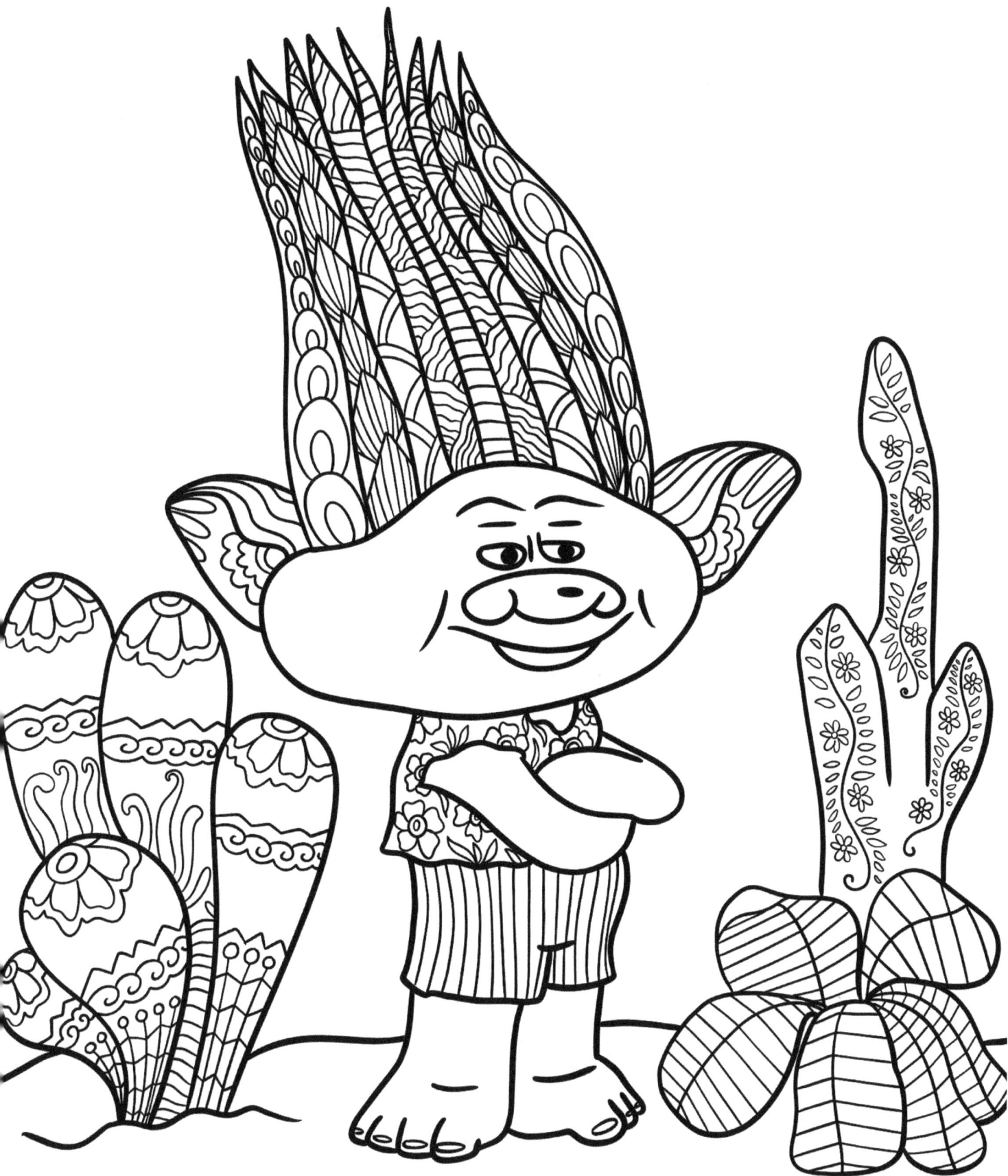

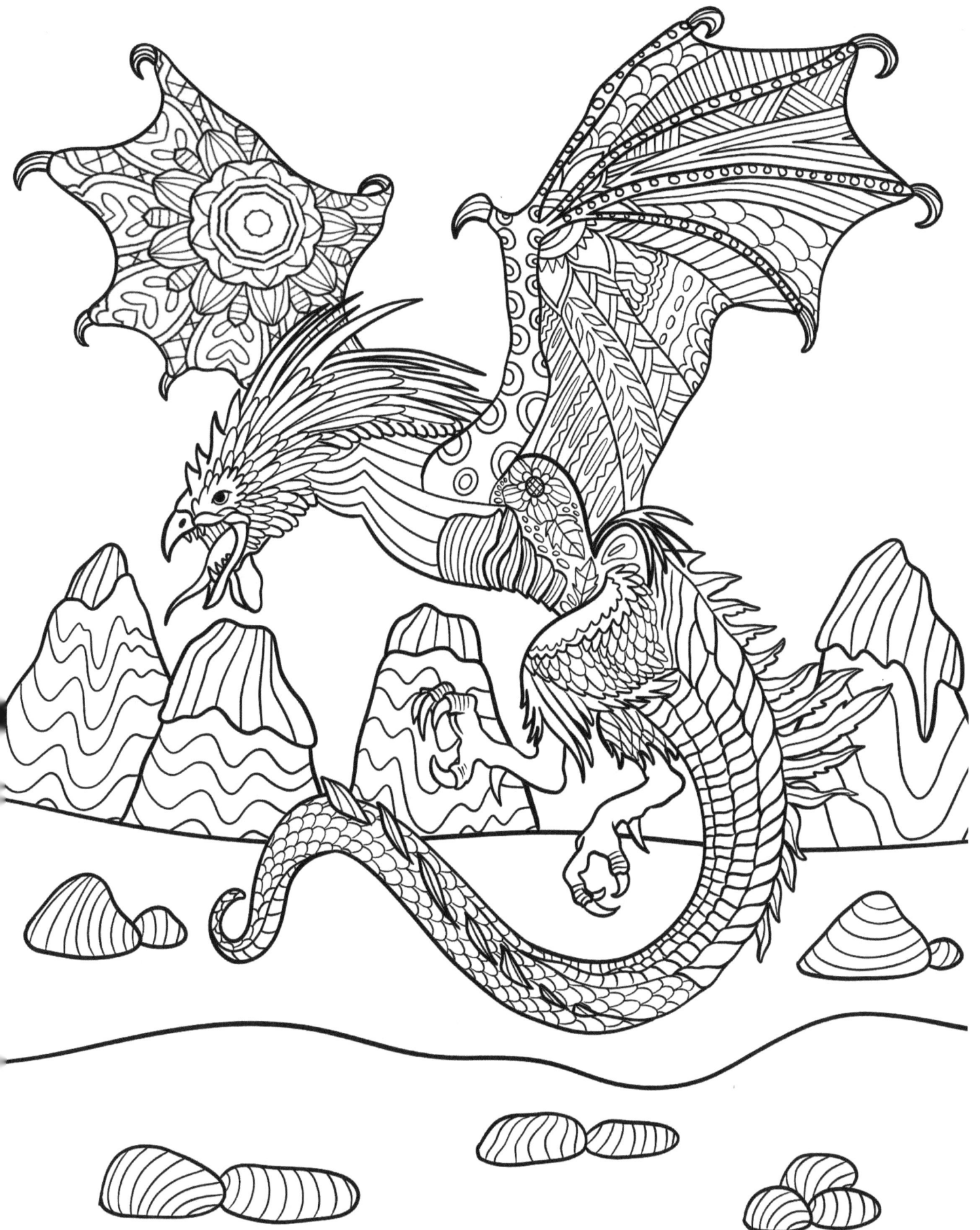

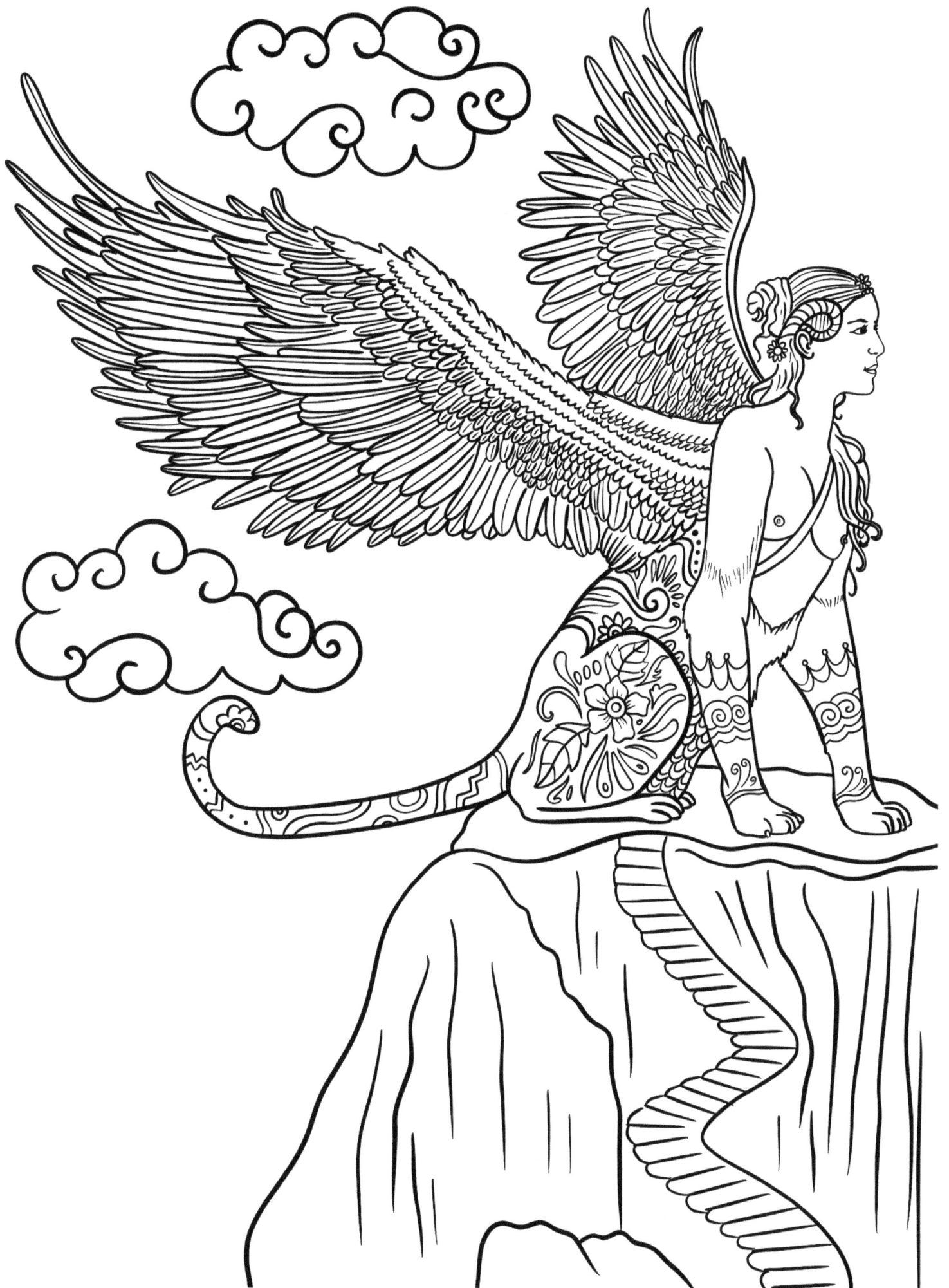

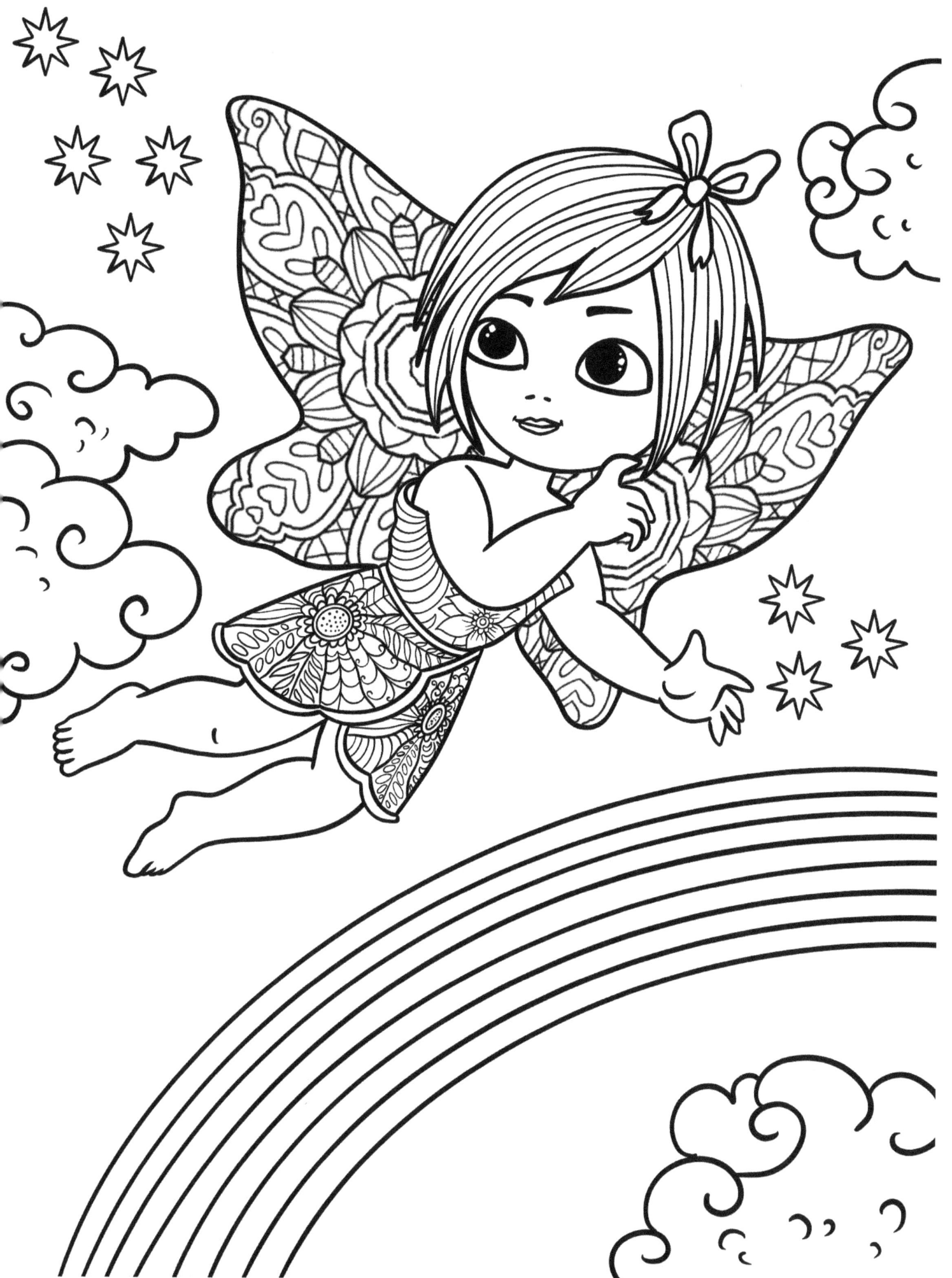

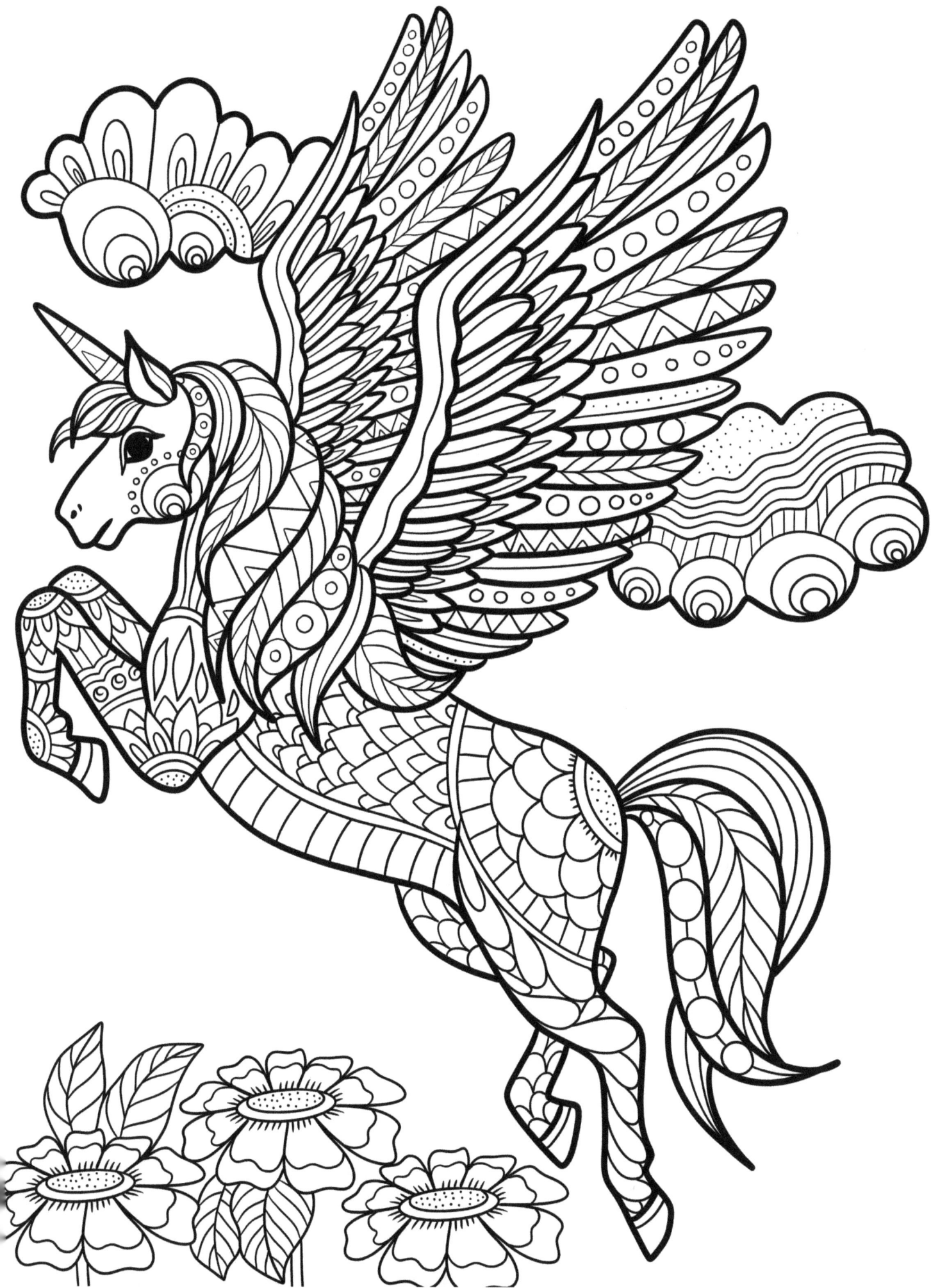

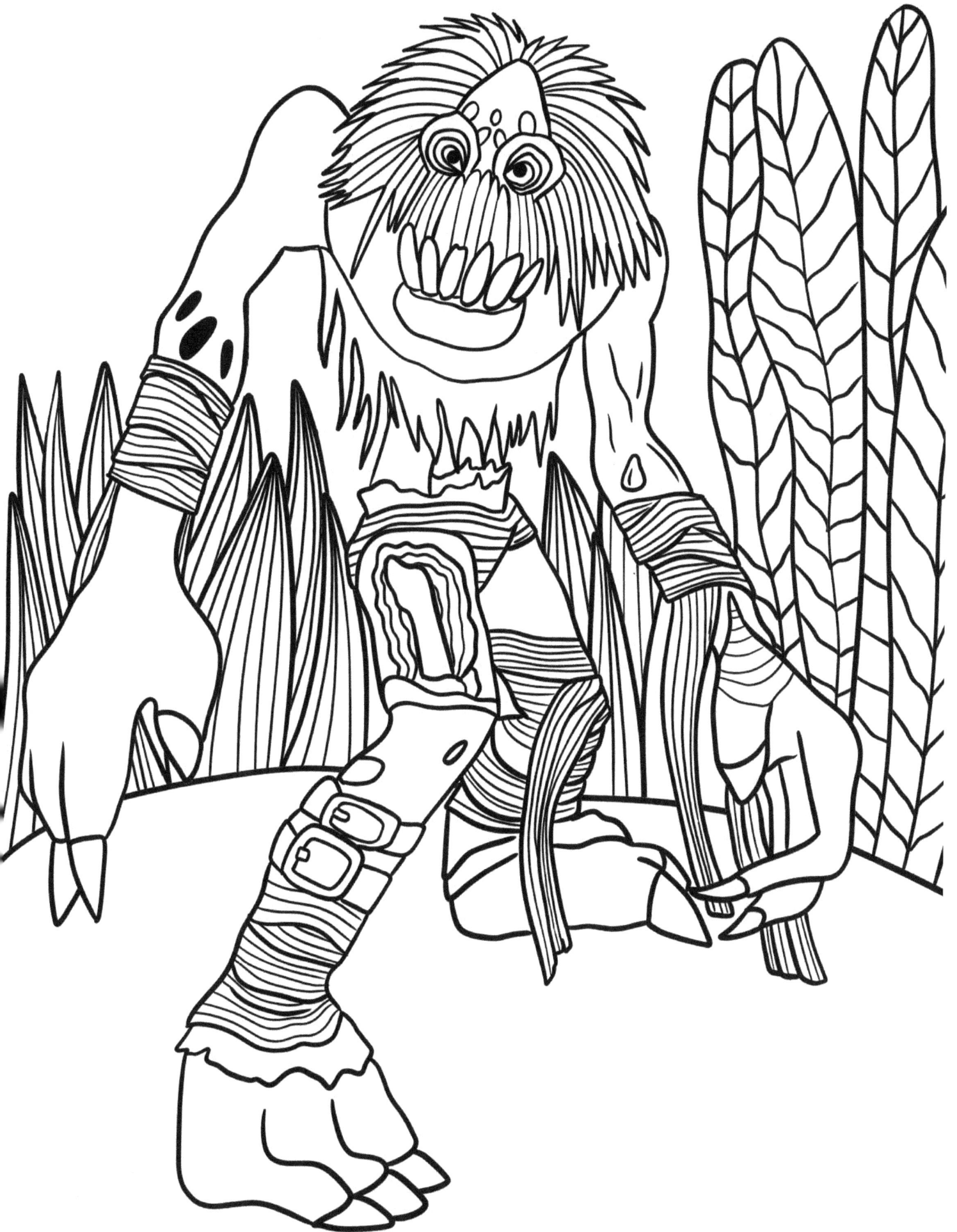

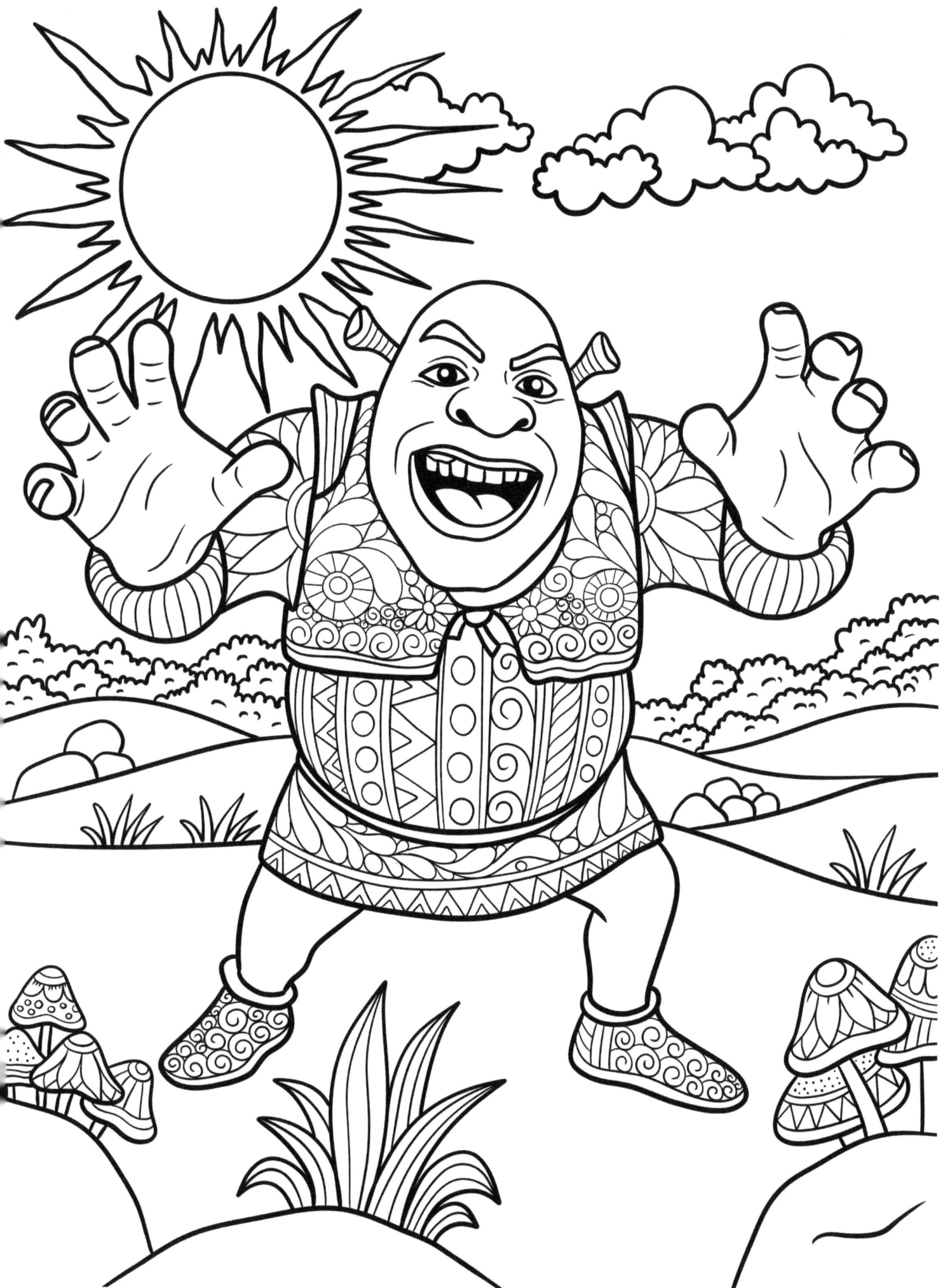

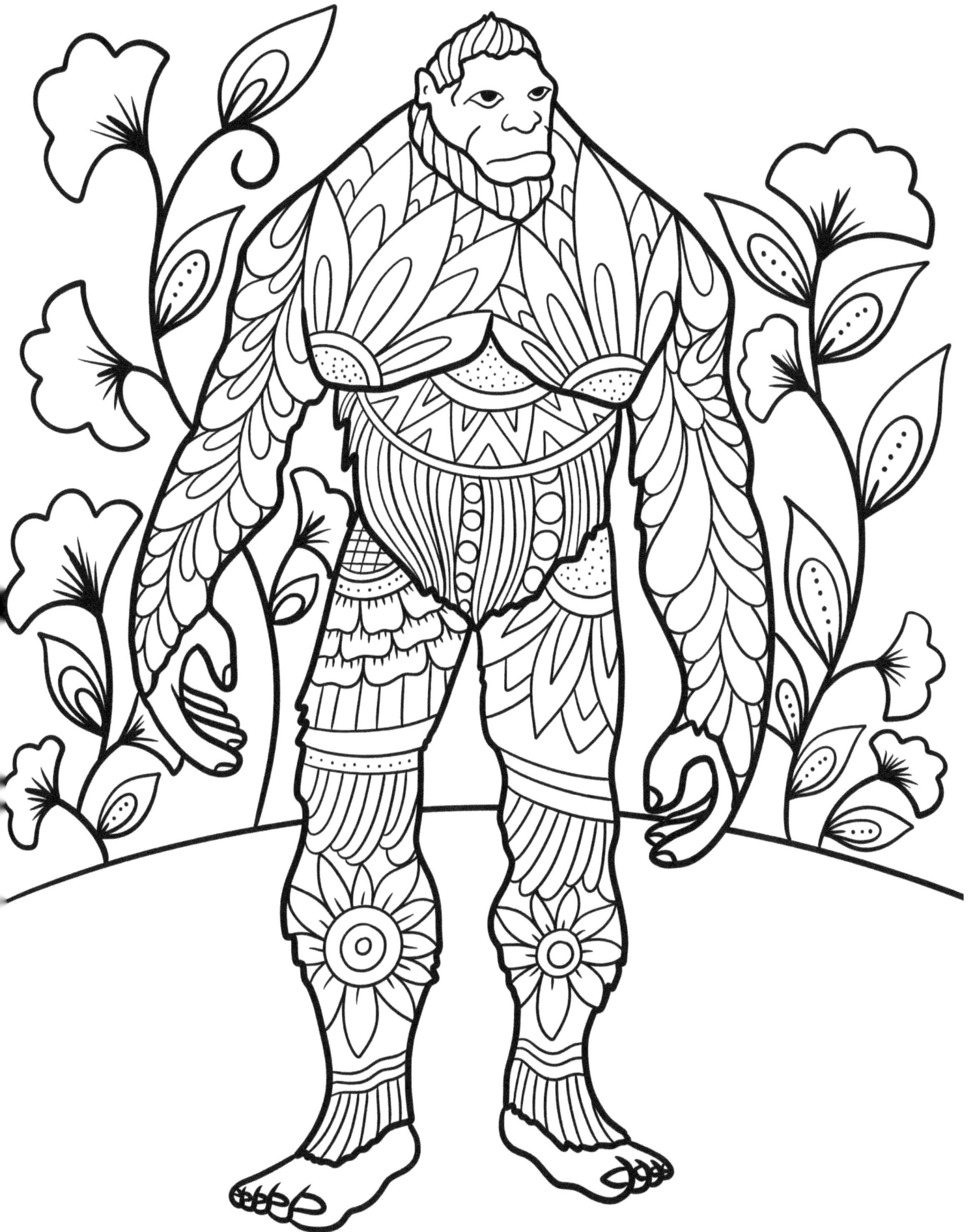

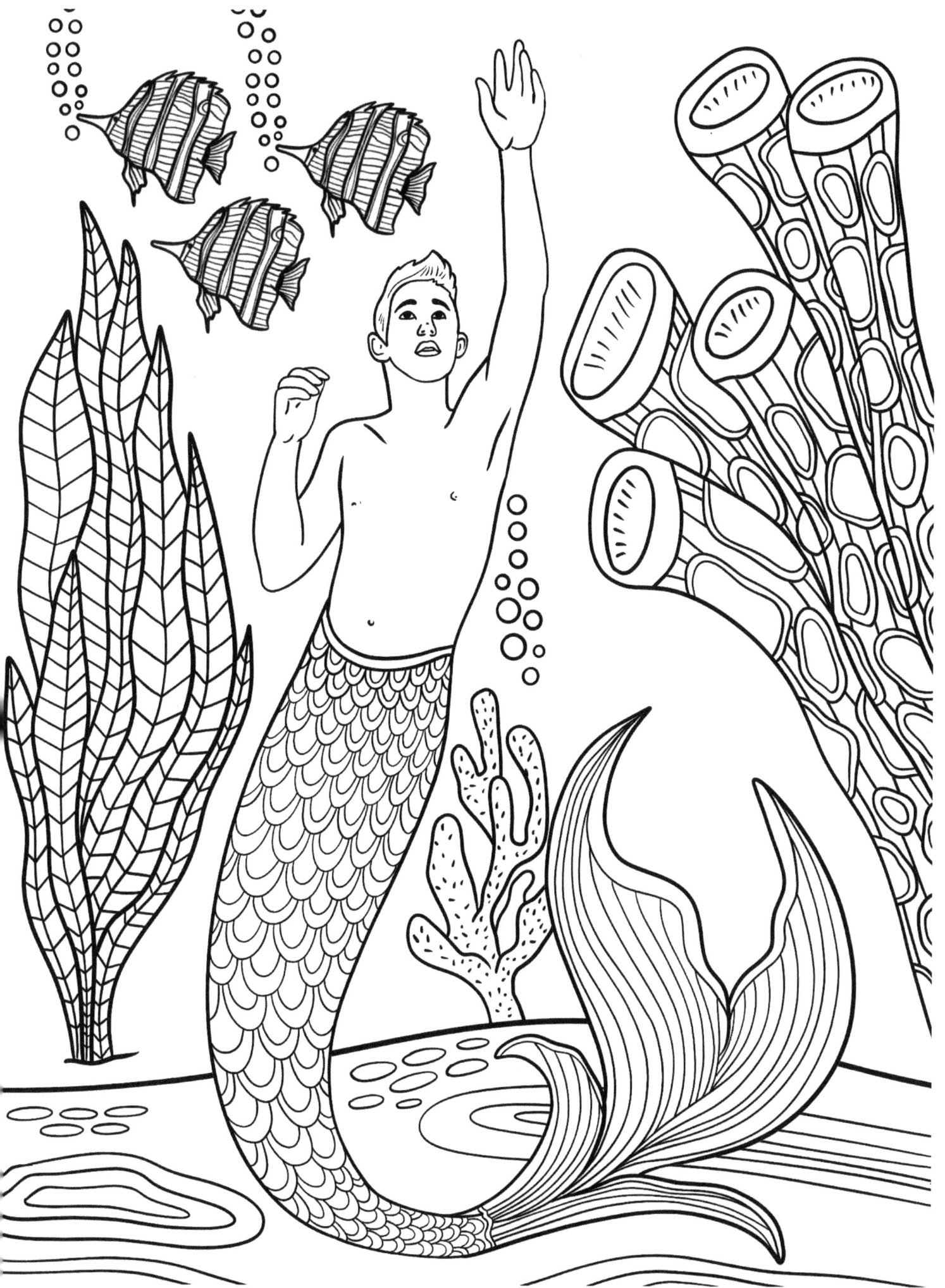

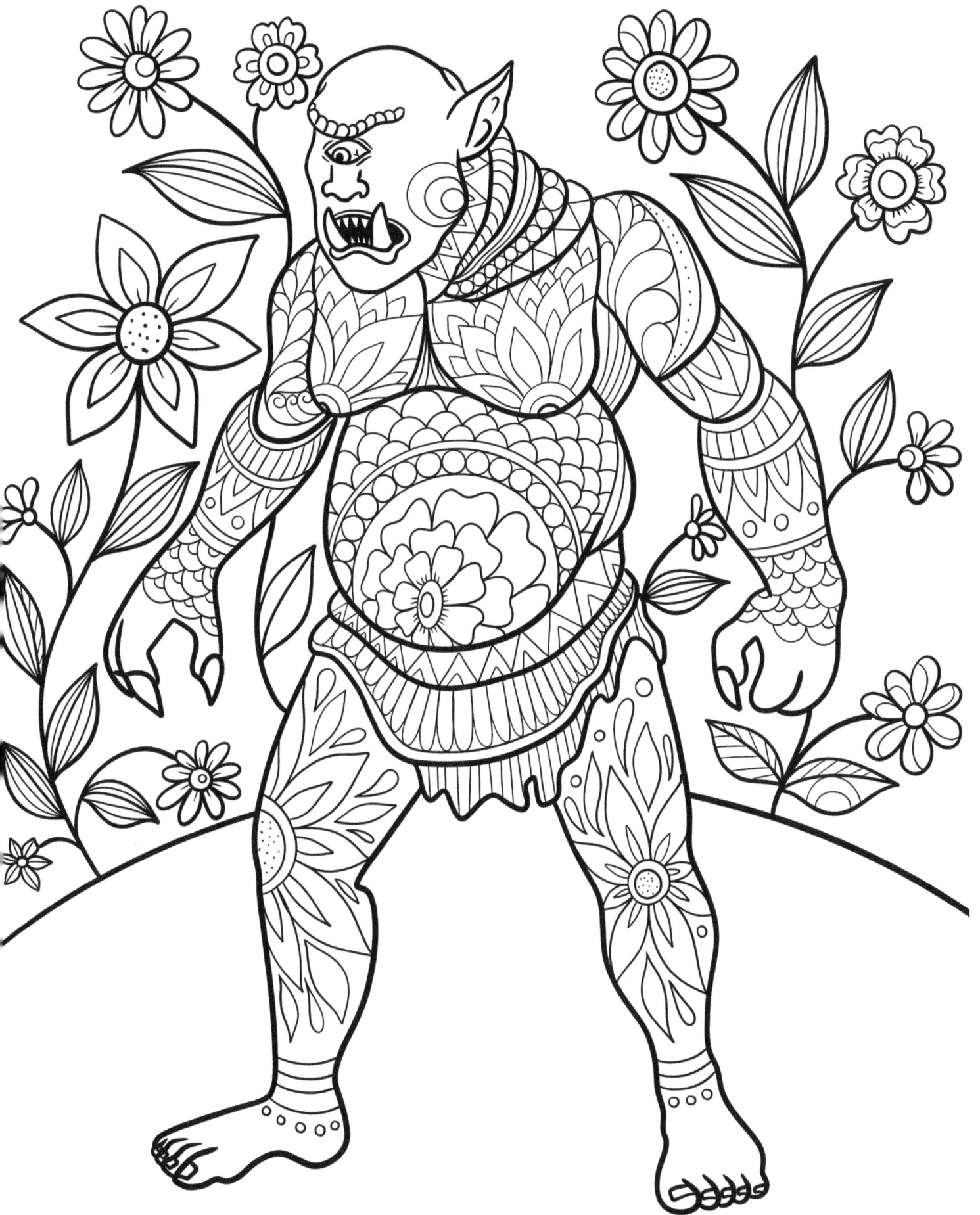

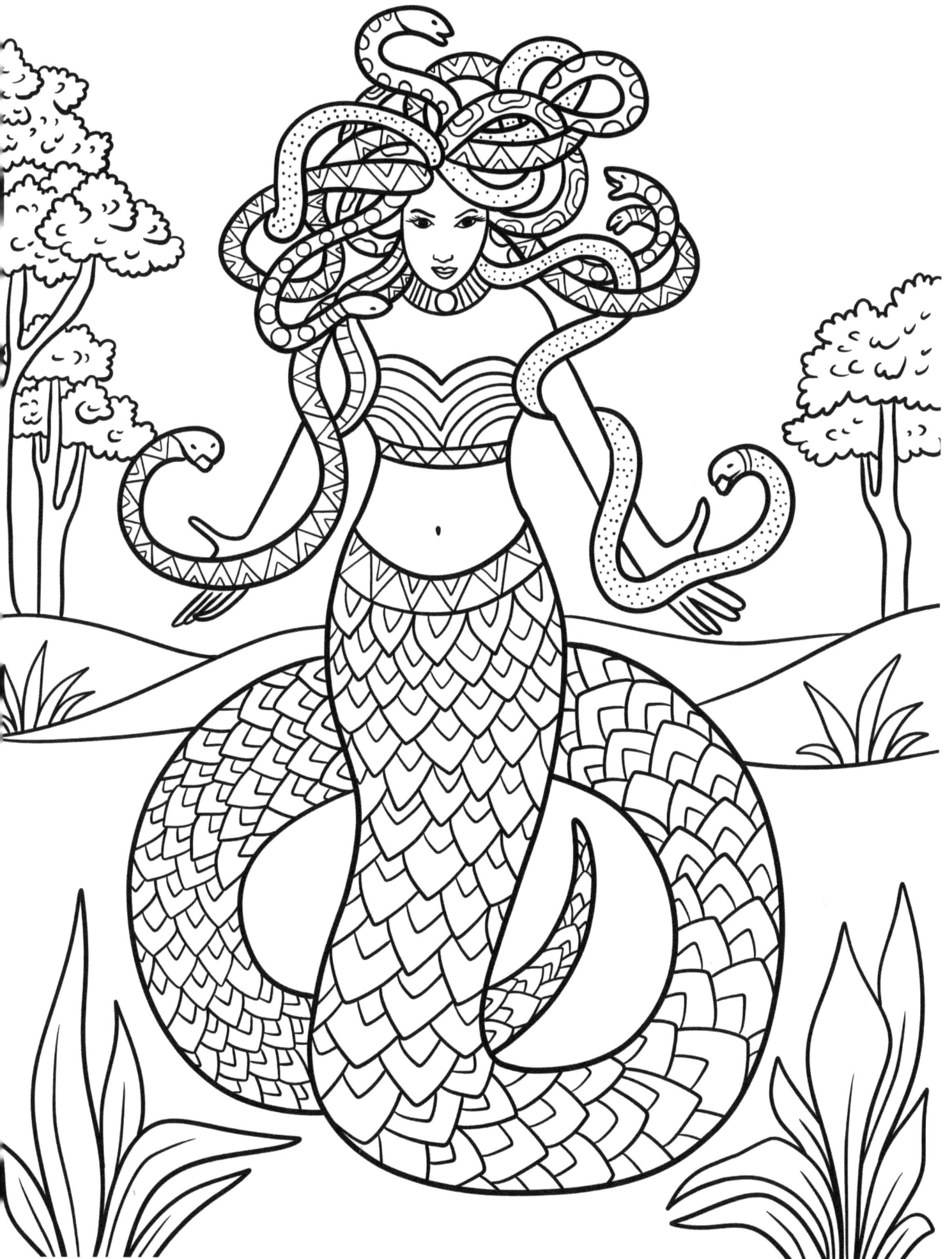

Thank you for purchasing this book.

If you would like to know more about Aryla Publishing Books please visit:-

www.ArylaPublishing.com

Or follow us on
Facebook
Twitter
Instagram
for *free promotions*

@arylapublishing

We would love to know what you think of this book so please leave us a review.

Have a wonderful day ☺

Other Coloring Books from Aryla Publishing

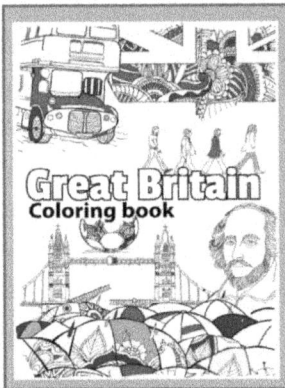

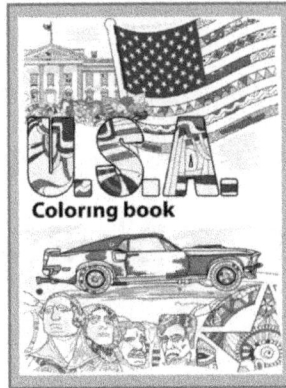

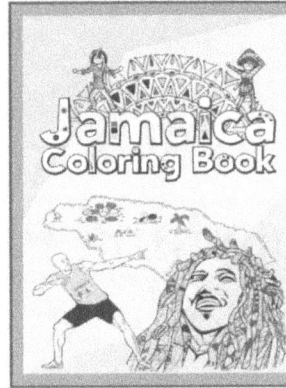

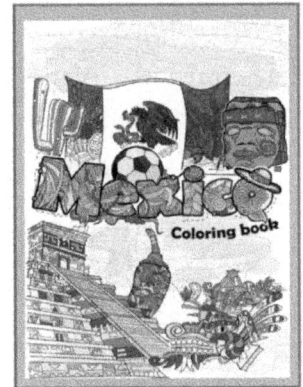

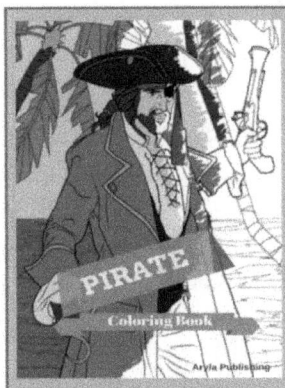

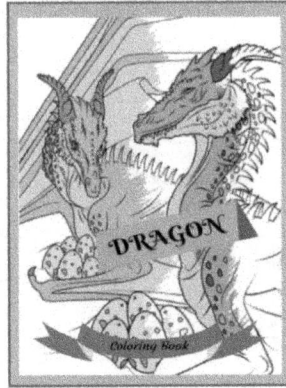

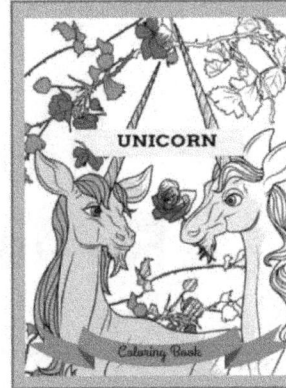

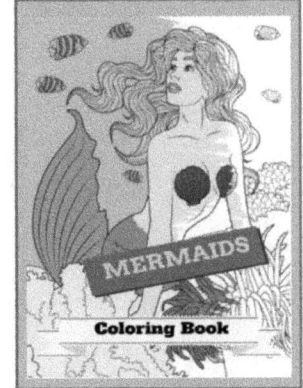

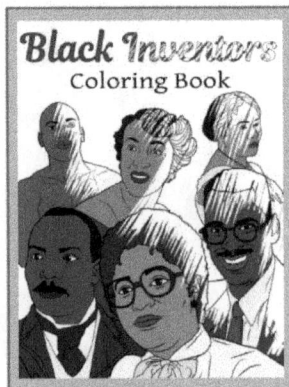

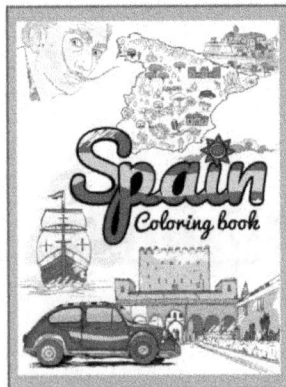

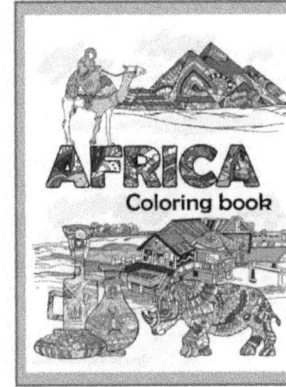

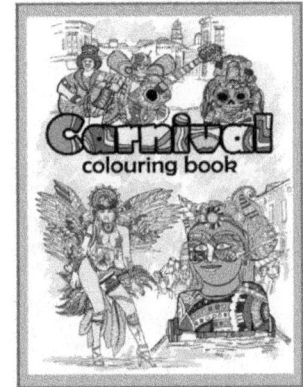

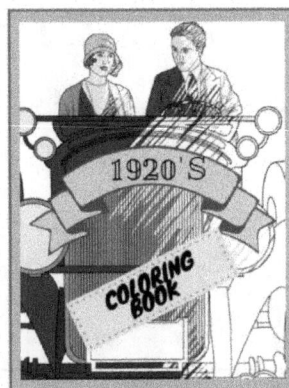

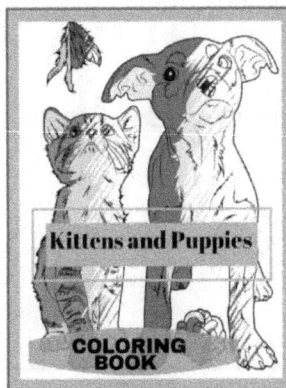

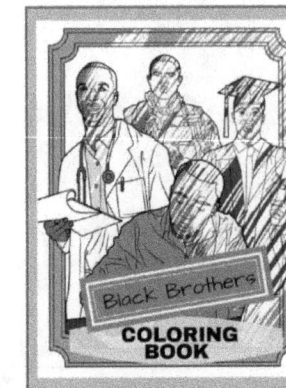

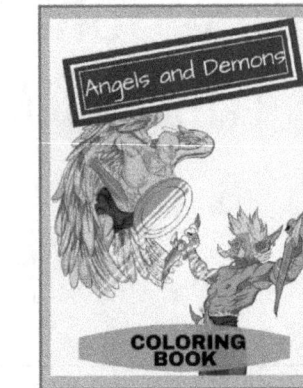

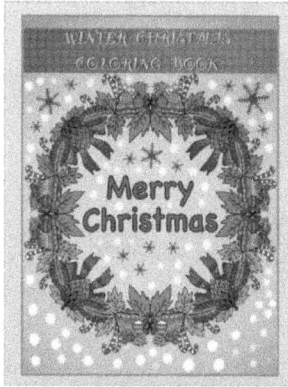
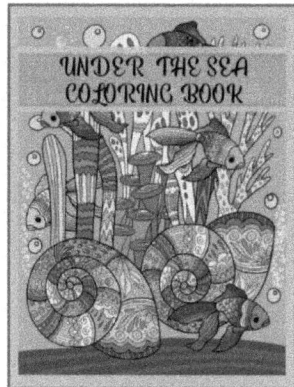
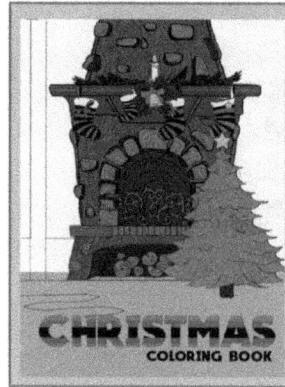
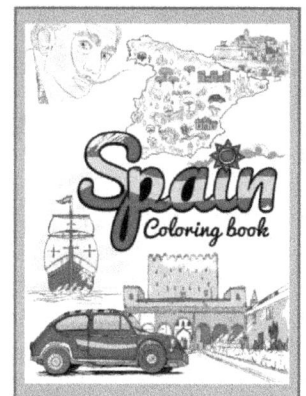
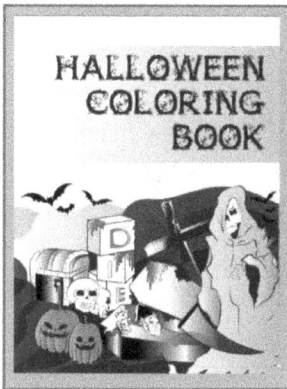
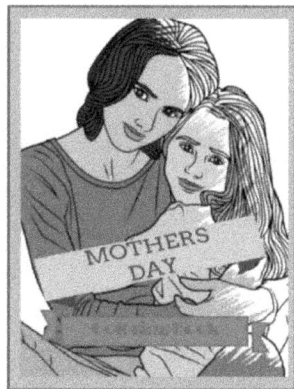
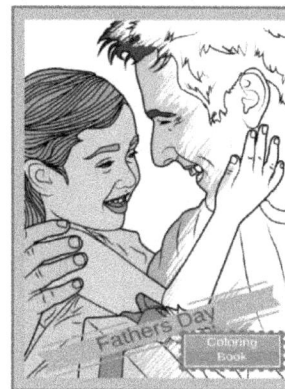
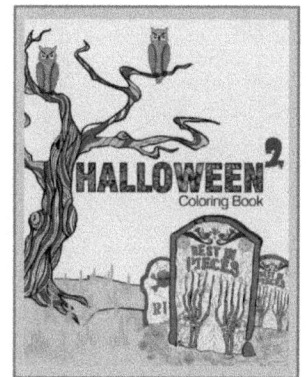
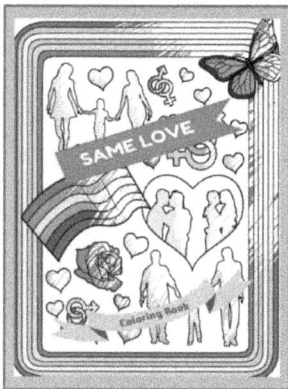
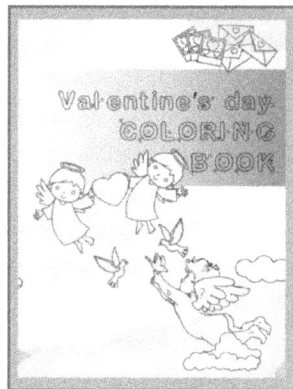
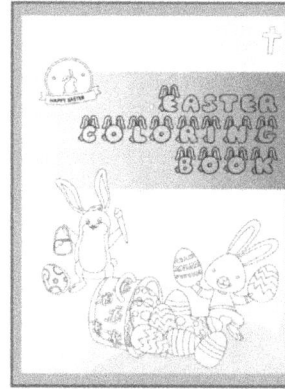
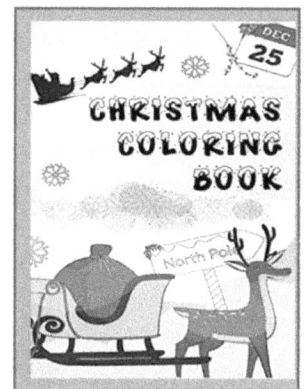
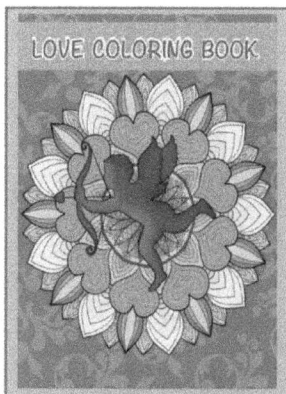
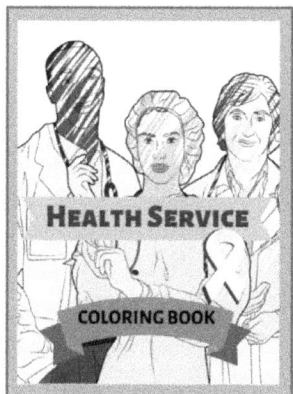
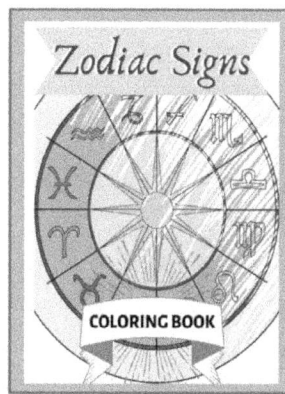
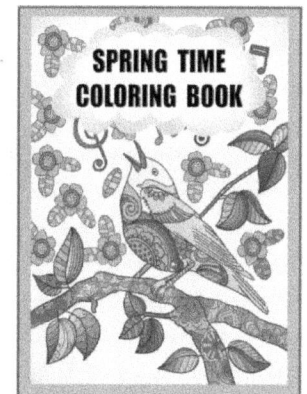

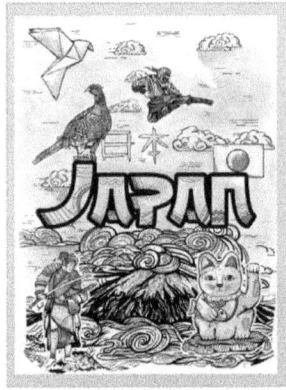

JAPAN

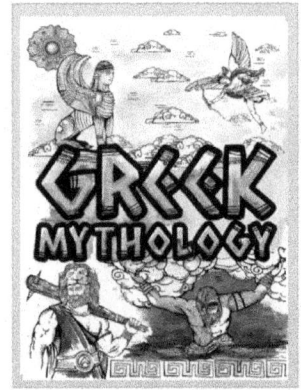

GREEK MYTHOLOGY

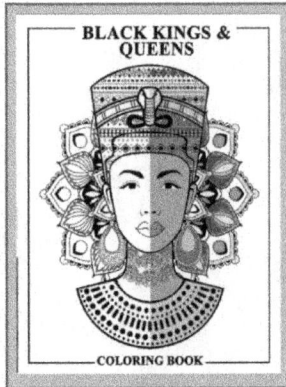

BLACK KINGS & QUEENS

COLORING BOOK

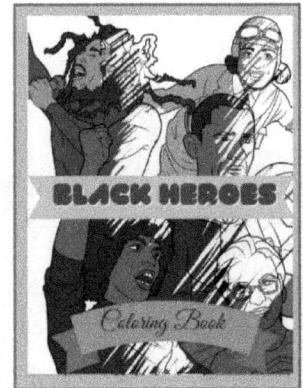

BLACK HEROES

Coloring Book

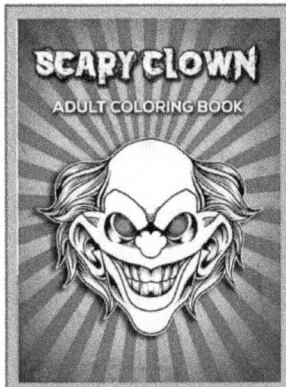

SCARY CLOWN

ADULT COLORING BOOK

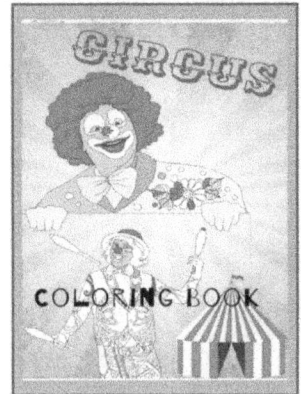

CIRCUS

COLORING BOOK

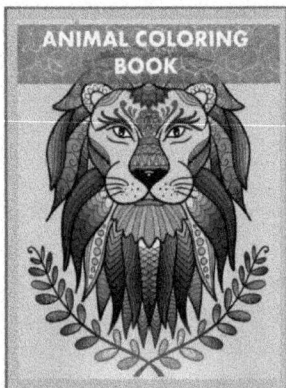

ANIMAL COLORING BOOK

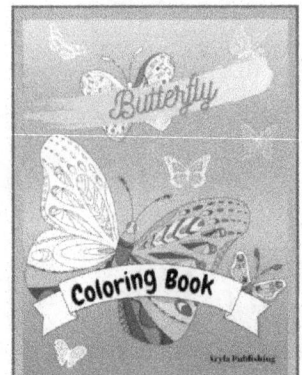

Butterfly

Coloring Book

Gryla Publishing

Color In Fun
Kids Books

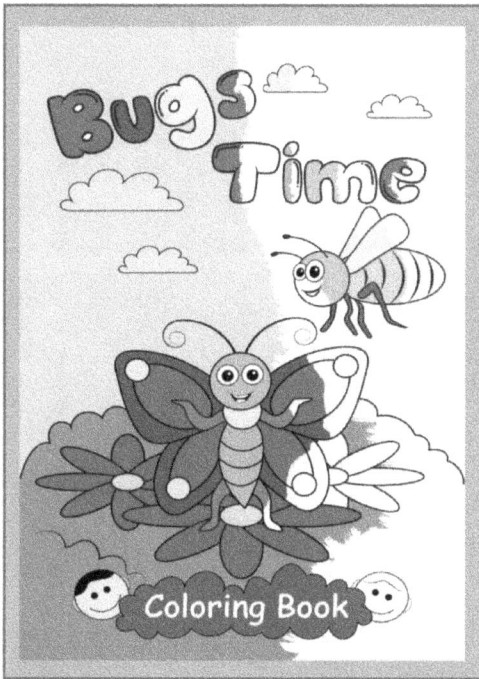

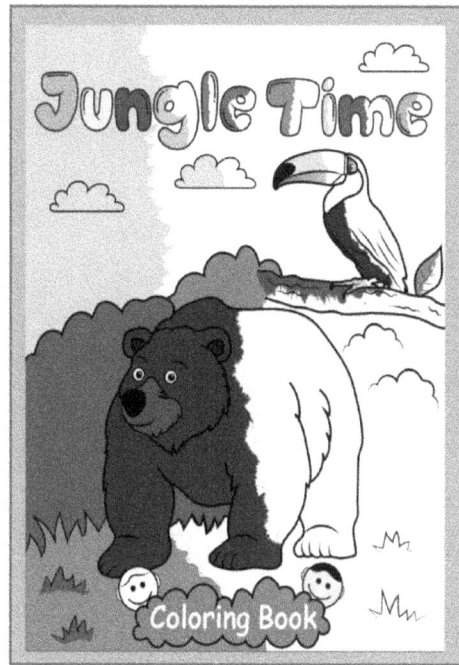

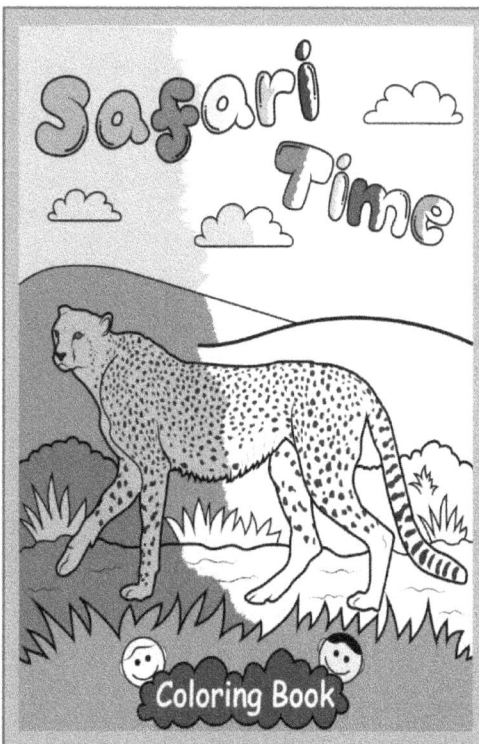

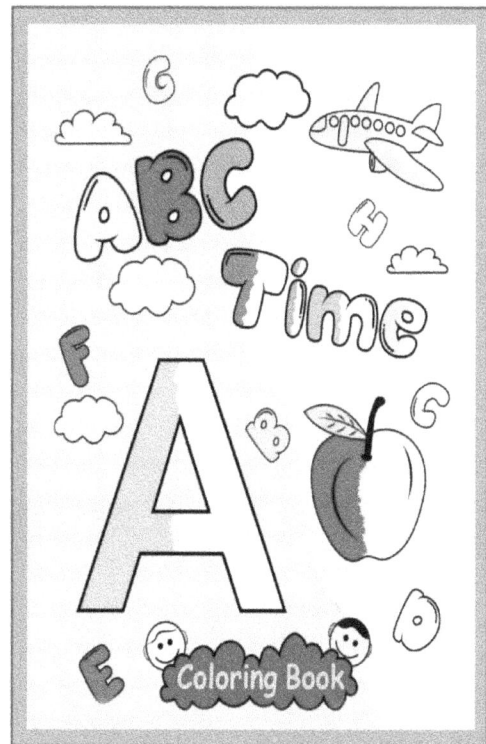

Bugs Time
Coloring Book

Jungle Time
Coloring Book

Safari Time
Coloring Book

ABC Time
Coloring Book

Visit **www.ArylaPublishing.com**

to find out about all new releases.

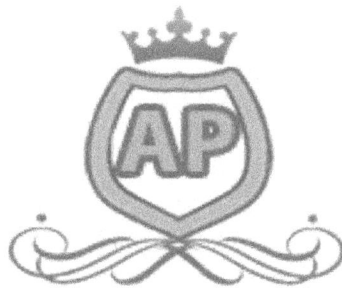

Follow us @arylapublishing on Twitter Instagram & Facebook

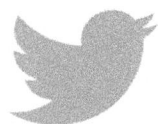

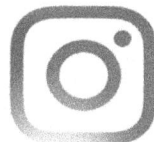

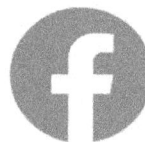

Search for Aryla Publishing on

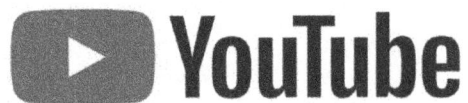

▶ **YouTube**

Check out our Book Trailers

Subscribe to keep up to date with new releases!

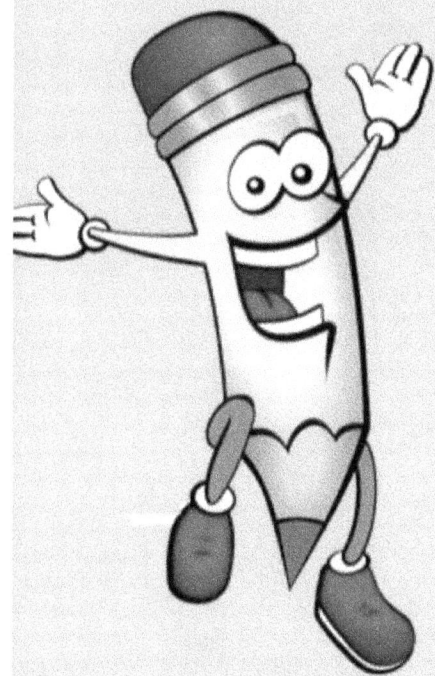

WE WOULD LOVE YOUR FEEDBACK

PLEASE LEAVE REVIEW AT:-

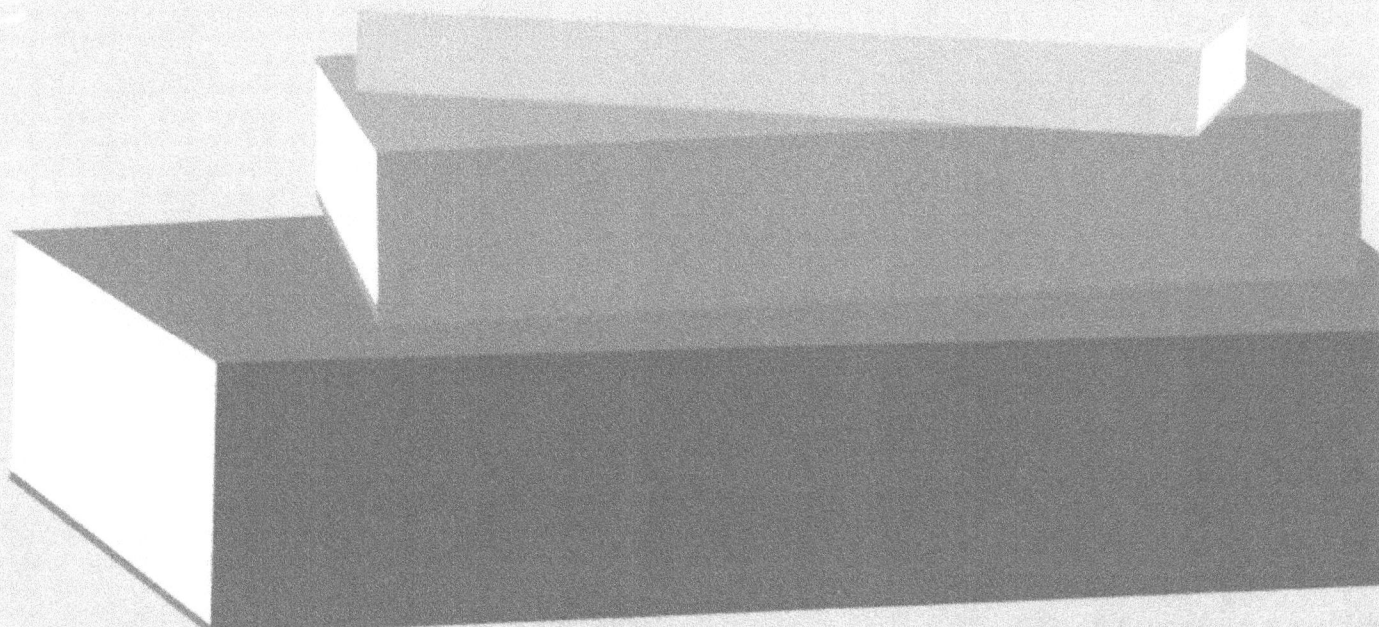

www.ingramcontent.com/pod-product-compliance
Lightning Source LLC
Chambersburg PA
CBHW081721270326
41933CB00017B/3250